SENIOR PROM

SENIOR PROM

◆

How Survivors of Long Marriages
Can Successfully Find
New Partners

Pat Hutchins

iUniverse, Inc.
New York Lincoln Shanghai

SENIOR PROM
How Survivors of Long Marriages Can Successfully Find New Partners

Copyright © 2007 by Patricia Hutchins

All rights reserved. No part of this book may be used or reproduced by any means, graphic, electronic, or mechanical, including photocopying, recording, taping or by any information storage retrieval system without the written permission of the publisher except in the case of brief quotations embodied in critical articles and reviews.

iUniverse books may be ordered through booksellers or by contacting:

iUniverse
2021 Pine Lake Road, Suite 100
Lincoln, NE 68512
www.iuniverse.com
1-800-Authors (1-800-288-4677)

Because of the dynamic nature of the Internet, any Web addresses or links contained in this book may have changed since publication and may no longer be valid.

You should not undertake any diet/exercise regimen recommended in this book before consulting your personal physician. Neither the author nor the publisher shall be responsible or liable for any loss or damage allegedly arising as a consequence of your use or application of any information or suggestions contained in this book.

ISBN: 978-0-595-43825-9 (pbk)
ISBN: 978-0-595-68376-5 (cloth)
ISBN: 978-0-595-88151-2 (ebk)

Printed in the United States of America

For Deborah, Lucy, Ross, and Martha Hutchins, as well Casey, Robert, Martha, Olivia, Alexandra, and Savanna, whose mother and grandmother I am.

For help along the way, I want to thank Roger Hutchins for big encouragement with my first computer, and particularly Ron Mueller for his extensive work on my manuscript, Alisa Aiken, Emilie Walker, and Leslie Waller for their excellent suggestions and much-valued time and generosity. And to daughter Deb who taught me the proper use of a semi-colon.

Some of the book's characters and their stories are pure fiction, used to illustrate a certain point I wished to make, and, as such, do not reflect situations or persons known to me.

In her mid-fifties Pat was on the staff of Manoir Westmount, a smart residence for lively and basically healthy retired men and women in an upscale area of Montreal.

Today, Pat lives on the north shore of Lake Erie, in Canada's Niagara Peninsula. You may contact her by e-mail: pathutchinscanada@hotmail.com.

Contents

Prologue 1

How and Where to Meet the Best New People: Part One

Chapter 1 Reclaim Your Life ... at sea in a single-again social climate you no longer recognize: a useable fail-safe plan is needed. 9

Chapter 2 Give Talent a Chance ... how to be part of the creative community in your city. 13

Chapter 3 How to Jump-start Your New Single-again Social Life ... activities with exciting possibilities. 17

Chapter 4 Shyness Is Not a Good Enough Reason ... how to find the perfect interest group that meets on a regular basis. 22

Chapter 5 A Man Talks to a Woman on the Move ... the art and reason to travel alone. 29

Chapter 6 A Widow Makes It on Her Own ... a dependent woman determinedly and delightfully regains independence. 33

Chapter 7 Three New Beginnings ... how three seasoned singles created their own employment to discover romance along the way. 38

Chapter 8 Shake Up Your Chances for Romance ... don't settle for dull. 46

Chapter 9	Take the "A" Train ... enjoy a luxury ride across the country with interesting friends you haven't yet met.	53
Chapter 10	Fresh Places to Look for New Friends ... unlikely places to find likely mates.	57
Chapter 11	Meeting In Person After Meeting Online ... play it responsibly, and play fairly.	62
Chapter 12	When You've Been Alone Too Long ... a proactive approach to better the odds.	67
Chapter 13	A Great Quiz for Both Men and Women ... to test your derring-do as a single-again adult.	69

Zero in on Problems that Need Fixing: Part Two

Chapter 14	Let's Get a Few Problems Out of the Way ... irritating habits from an old relationship gotta go!	73
Chapter 15	Solitude Has Its Advantages ... it takes guts to rejoin life: with one small step you can do it!	79
Chapter 16	You Asked Him Out How Many Times? Maybe he's just not that interested.	82
Chapter 17	Facing Up to Alcoholism ... one woman's story of increased alcohol dependency after her divorce; her victory over bitterness.	87
Chapter 18	For Men Only ... get-with-it dating 101.	100
Chapter 19	Didn't Plan on Being Poor at Seventy ... how two smart widows solved their money worries.	102
Chapter 20	Screw Impotence! Just choose the right partner and quit your worry ... strong facts on limp members.	106
Chapter 21	Time to Toss Drunks, Married Lovers, Liars, and Moody Jerks ... you don't need any of them.	109

Chapter 22   Never Let Yourself Be Degraded ... anyone is not better than no one if that person is ignorant of your feelings. 115

Chapter 23   He Didn't See Her Coming ... a vulnerable man falls for a female con. 117

Chapter 24   Grown Children Angry Over Their Parents' Divorce ... your divorce wasn't their idea, don't look for their sympathy. 120

Chapter 25   Concerning "Formers" and "Exes" ... and why to keep your mouth shut about them. 124

Chapter 26   When Your Lover Exhibits a Violent Temper ... be very clear on this: do not hesitate to walk away. 126

Chapter 27   Your First Date In Years ... and it could be your last if you do nothing but fire off a battery of questions.. 130

Chapter 28   The Angry Child You Could Inherit ... a no-nonsense face-off with your new partner's upset adult child.. 133

Your Healthy Attitude is Key: Part Three

Chapter 29   Get Body Smart ... on top of the world with new energy. 139

Chapter 30   Perking Up Brain Activity ... the brain can and will continue to rewire and adapt as it ages: it starts with reading. 144

Chapter 31   Two Quick No-Cook Soups (from a non-cook). ... 147

Chapter 32   Stress Got You? Give physical and emotional tension the boot! 150

Chapter 33   Safety Inside Your Home ... tips from the Council on Aging. 156

Chapter 34	Street Smarts ... face the streets with confidence. ...	160
Chapter 35	Thieves of Comfort: anger, arthritis, adult hearing loss, and sleeplessness.	163
Chapter 36	Dating After a Mastectomy ... a tribute to real men, as well a huge cheer to my mother, Audrey Safford Orr, and to author Barbara Delinsky.	169
Chapter 37	To Share a Bedroom or Not ... the case for 2 bedrooms with intriguing visiting privileges.	171

Perfecting your Hidden Skills: Part Four

Chapter 38	The Fear Factors ... identify and specify valid fears to find informed answers.	175
Chapter 39	Stand Up for Yourself ... there's something impeccably boring about a totally accommodating man or woman.	178
Chapter 40	Take Good Care of Friendship ... a good friend can outlast a slew of husbands.	181
Chapter 41	A Man Finds His Lost Love ... the indelible woman he never forgot.	182
Chapter 42	How to Get Invited to Parties ... first you give a party to remember!	199
Chapter 43	Find Your Personal Neighborhood Escape Hatch ... when you can't stand your own company.	201
Chapter 44	Home Stagers ... an all-round winner of a job in house showcasing—and you don't need a graduate degree.	204
Chapter 45	Expand Your World With Computer Savvy ... upgrade your skills and abilities.	207

Chapter 46 Flattery Is a Win-Win Situation ... any woman who understands how to flatter men has heaps more fun!! 210

Grooming for all your Fabulous Tomorrows: Part Five

Chapter 47 Who Said Younger Is Better? (For Women Only) ... relaxed and natural is what really attracts men...... 215

Chapter 48 Who Said Younger Is Better? (For Men Only) ... self-confidence is what really attracts women........ 218

Chapter 49 Bald and Faking It ... pleeeze quit it!............. 221

Chapter 50 Behind Closed Doors ... always your best personal grooming habits............................. 222

Bring it on! You're Ready for a Brilliant Future: Part Six

Chapter 51 A Mate-Selection Quiz for Late Lovers ... designed to make you think—definitely not a first date test paper..................................... 227

Chapter 52 Goodbye Loneliness, Hello Happiness ... open yourself optimistically to new experiences with unexpected people........................... 233

Bibliography *237*

Prologue

What made me notice her was she looked so entirely out of place, as if she'd been stuck in the wrong spot on the wrong plane. Her very oddness got my attention, and I kept my eye on her erratic progress down the aisle between the cushy seats of first class. She passed the dividing curtain shielding moneyed from budget-conscious travelers and kept coming toward me through the densely packed tourist section, bumping a hip, then an elbow on tall seat backs and catching her shoe on sticking out pieces of carry-on luggage as she checked every few rows to get her bearings. She carried a disheveled mess of plastic shopping bags, purses, and a shoulder-slung camera, and somehow I just knew she was headed for the empty seat beside me.

By the time she came to an abrupt halt and squinted at the numbers on the rack above my seat row, she looked totally undone. I smiled up at her worn face and jammed my carry-on another inch farther under my seat so she could settle in. She eyed her allotted space suspiciously, "Good thing for both of us I'm a skinny one," she muttered.

Her blue plastic-rimmed glasses were cocked toward her right ear, and a single silver hairpin hung uselessly from a Frenchy arrangement of white hair at the nape of her neck. "It's so difficult to travel alone, and everyone seems to be in such a hurry and kind of cross with me," her shaky voice almost broke as she tugged at her lap belt. She managed a shy smile. "I tell you, I think I'm on the Lord's shit list!"

My eyebrows shot up. Instantly she said, "I'm Eudora, but friends call me Dorit, and I'm a widow. Four months ago, that's when he went. One day he's there, and then next thing you know he's gone! I'll never forgive the dirty bugger for leaving me on my own." I started to laugh. I liked her.

She knew it, and cannily elected me confessor of her fears and heartache. As she picked up speed, her words ran together in a litany of her deceased husband Joe's deeds and misdeeds of forty-four years; even before the plane had reached cruising altitude, I likely knew more about Joe than his own mother knew in her entire lifetime.

She was adorable, but she just couldn't shut up. She was full of wonderful stories of happier times, and she delighted in telling all. And I do mean all!

"The minute I laid eyes on that devil, I knew he was my man—the way he walked, tall and loose, and the way he looked at me kinda saucy-like through eyes that weren't all the way open. You ever have a guy look at you like that, you grab him fast. It's what they call bedroom eyes, and I tell you straight, I almost went blind in his bedroom at Seward's rooming house for the next few months till my father cornered him one day on Main Street in front of Peck's drugstore and told him, 'Sonny, you make an honest woman outta my little girl, or I'm gonna run you clean outta town.'"

If she talked like that to me, a perfect stranger, I can only imagine what more she told close friends. Nothing stood in her way as she delivered an unending monologue on her freshly dead husband and the fact that she loved and missed him so much that all she wanted was to find another husband immediately. At that very moment I was set to send the mythical husband a muzzle for her mouth as a wedding gift. Dorit had a true problem. It wasn't just her marathon mouth; her problem was she was overwhelmed with loneliness. If it was hard on her, it was also hard on people around her awash in her unstoppable talk.

In Florida, where I live, there's a large population of retired people who find the year-round climate appealing. Inevitably some of those thousands of married men and women will find themselves alone again. It happens after the death, or divorce, of a mate in marriages that have often survived for decades. No matter the cause, when it happens, the emptiness can be nearly unbearable.

Dorit wasn't being disloyal to Joe or to his memory because she wanted to remarry immediately. In her own fashion, she was complimenting him. She'd loved being married. She wanted to continue that kind of a life, but she hadn't the faintest idea how she was going to make it happen. If she didn't learn to shut up occasionally, any potential new husband would keel over, cross-eyed from exhaustion, before she ever got him to the altar. My mind was reeling with much more information than I could handle comfortably after only thirty minutes in her company: strung together stories of Dorit and Joe's adventures, joys, losses, successes, and failures. Eventually she ran out of steam and fell asleep in the middle of a sentence.

She was a very pretty woman when her tension eased and her face relaxed. I watched her face in repose with a mixture of sadness and relief; when the drinks cart went by I quickly told the flight attendant that Dorit wasn't at all thirsty, but I'd like a double of whatever they had the most of.

Flying smoothly above the clouds, I reclined my seat and closed my eyes. I thought about the thousands of lonely men and women who are left to manage on their own after longtime marriages or long-standing love affairs are over. My mind scrolled through a list of friends who were left alone when a wife or husband of many years died or wanted out of the marriage. The list grew longer every year. I thought of my neighbor, Sam, and his appalling struggle with his beautiful Sarah, a victim of Alzheimer's disease, unable to do a damned thing while he watched everything that particularized his wife's personality slowly fade and eventually disappear. The two had met in a life drawing class at art school thirty years earlier. He found it so very hard to be on his own again after her death.

There was Richard, shattered by a separation coming at a time when least expected. I ran into him at a party a couple of weeks after his wife filed for divorce. "What in hell does Helen mean," he yelled at me (he's very deaf and always refuses to wear his hearing aide), "that I'm not the man she married? She married me forty years ago, for gawdsake. Of course I'm not the same man!"

And Millie, too, after forty-five years with Oscar, felt the cruel blow that many long-term wives dread. Her husband found a much younger woman who, in turn, found Oscar witty and exciting, and happily became his hedge against dodderiness. The fact that he was gigantically rich hadn't hurt his appeal. Oscar reacted in typical fashion—he sucked in his stomach and avoided discussing his life before the birth of computers. Millie, at sixty-four years of age, says there are no good men around. She's wrong. She's just not looking in the right places.

My own marriage, after some twenty years, had ended sadly in divorce, and I was on my own again with four teenagers when I was in my early forties. It was difficult enough at that age to regain my sense of self. Understandably it's a great deal more difficult for even older men and women to start over again and make sense of their lives at an age when one isn't as flexible in handling major change. Which is exactly why, these many years later, as a happily confident woman with a full social life, a grown family, and a seriously delirious lover, I wanted to write this book with sound, useable tips for men and women who are alone again after long-time marriages or partnerships are over. It's a practical guide on how to succeed as an older person returning to the current world of dating, interpersonal relations, and single life.

Survivors of long-time marriages need help to find another partner. Before that, however, they need some help to clean up their acts so that a new partnership starts on strong footing. There are plenty of lonely men and women who, like Dorit (thankfully still sweetly asleep beside me in seat 32B), feel totally at sea with a single-again life they hadn't asked for.

This group of older singles is huge. The numbers run too high to be ignored. In the year 2005 there were 10,934,000 men and women over sixty-five living alone in the U.S., an increase of 1,750,000 single and single-again men and women in that age group since year 1997 **(from the statistical abstract of the United States Bureau of the Census).**

These are not single people living within families, or in institutions; the figures reflect persons living independently. The huge numbers of persons over sixty-five living alone indicate, in the main, a population that was once married and living in partnership. There's another alarming figure of 15,220,000 American men and women over sixty-five living alone projected for the year 2020. By the year 2030 there are projected to be 50 million men and women, that is 73% of the gross population of people over sixty-five in The United States, who will be singles. The fact of their single-again lives is for the most part not one of choice.

Statistics Canada (Statistiques Canada) year 2007 published data reports that the most profound impact on Canada's demographics is the Baby-Boomers born in the two decades after the Second World War. By year 2016 (at the latest) Canada will have far more seniors than children under the age of fourteen, a phenomenon never before recorded in the country's history. The singles population at that time is projected at 70 percent of the gross population of that age group. Interesting to note that because of narrowing gender mortality differences, men are steadily gaining ground to match life expectancy of their female counterparts. When we reach year 2026, one out of every five people in Canada will be a senior.

If you're alone again after years with the same mate, you do not have to be alone forever. If you feel ready to find new love now, this book can show you how to make it happen.

Senior Prom is a positive look at finding new love after an old love is gone. With it, you can go from despair to hope, from lonely to complete, from single to couple. You'll grin again. Anyone who has lost a partner of many years will gain insight and courage as well as a practical plan of action to follow to find his or her best self, and then, to find another love.

Understandably, just the idea of taking that first scary step can nail you to the spot. The first step (more like a big shove!) is to stop staring at the past. Your next move is to jump into the ring and risk another chance at happiness.

For any single-again woman or man between fifty and ninety who wants to find a new partner, this is a book that can make you a much happier person. Actually, not the book by itself—it can't do a thing for you. It's the application of the material in the book that can, if you let it, change your life and have you looking lively to the future. This book is your map to rev up your life and grab a new partner for the Senior Prom.

How and Where to Meet the Best New People: Part One

1

Reclaim Your Life

At the outset, no matter how strong you are, almost everyone who's alone again and lonely after losing a long-time partner is nervous about dating. What sane person wouldn't be? You'd almost have to be a dope *not* to be nervous.

Loved ones come and go in a lifetime, but the ability and the capacity to love remains. If you're divorced, if your spouse has died, if you are alone again after many years with one partner, you may feel it's too late to find another person to love. It's never too late.

Single and single-again women and men with fifty, sixty, seventy, eighty years behind them *can* start fresh with a new mate. All too often what holds people back is they haven't a clue as to how to get going. A fail-safe plan is needed: a plan of action, a clear straightforward path to follow to find a feel-good, lasting relationship.

Attitudes have changed considerably since your first go-around, and in the present social climate, you're no longer expected to accept the loss of a long-term partner and then set about the job of aging gracefully till you croak. Aging gracefully is almost too much to expect from anyone over eight years old. It's more fun, and certainly much healthier, to let go of old attitudes and move beyond self-set limits (or those imposed by overprotective family or friends) to find a new mate for a fresh start.

Late loves are the same as the early loves of your life in all the important areas. Perhaps not as agile, firm or impetuous, but the emotions are the same. Intelligence is deeper, patience has developed, wisdom is kinder: all the fine qualities have endured. There is a learned understanding that being loved is a huge and welcome bonus of loving, that falling in love means a whole lot more than finding a nice person; mostly all it takes is being a nice person. And *that*, you are already!

One of the biggest "single again" hurdles is learning to become emotionally self-reliant. For the present time anyway, there's no one around to shore you up when you're wavering, to listen to your worries and fears, to bolster your ego, to run interference in a family matter, or to help solve your problems.

It's frightening to find yourself alone after years of being protected. At times you're bound to be discouraged, but your situation can improve. It *can* be fixed. But just like anything else that requires change, you have to be willing to put in the work to build a new life that will be quite different from the one you knew as half of a married couple.

If you've neglected friends because of your spouse's lengthy illness or because of divorce headaches, you could be in for some surprises. Good friends will understand that you had a lot to cope with, and they'll be there for you. Some acquaintances will have filled the gap that you left in their lives with new activities and new people. Others won't want you around because it throws out the seating at their formal dinner parties. Don't try to figure that one out. Accept it. See it as an opportunity to rethink your current friendships. Maybe it's time to broaden your boundaries to include friends you haven't yet met.

You probably haven't socialized as a single person in a very long time and although it's not exactly like jumping without a parachute, it does promise to stir up some excitement. A rewarding start is to offer your services as a volunteer worker so you can see clearly how valued you are.

If your finances are secure and you don't have to earn income, there are scores of volunteer groups that need your help. Daytime volunteers are always needed, but the most sought after volunteer is someone who is willing to work nights and weekends. This can suit you perfectly (whether or not you have a paying job), if you live alone and find these times especially lonely. Hospital auxiliaries, for instance, operate on a year-round day and evening schedule, and I know from my own volunteer experience that it's hard to get volunteers to work with patients on a Sunday. Most hospitals have a volunteer office within the hospital; a phone call can get you an appointment for an interview.

If you've spent too much time in hospitals recently and it's the last place on earth you want to be, there are plenty of other worthwhile groups that can use your help.

Museums and art galleries will train volunteer docents to be knowledgeable about artifacts and art so they can conduct paying visitors through the exhibits. You'll meet others, like yourself, who recognize the importance of keeping interest in the arts alive, plus you'll learn a lot of fascinating history in the process.

And there's the Humane Society, the symphony, the Institute for the Blind, the Red Cross, plus other deserving organizations that benefit abused children and battered spouses; they all need volunteers. And that's only skimming the list.

Through a public library literacy program you can teach an adult who hasn't had the opportunity for education, to read. It's a huge thrill to watch a person start to understand just what all those letters on the page mean. That kind of reward cannot be bought.

Amnesty International needs crucial assistance for people living under terrifying regimes and conditions we cannot begin to imagine. As well Americans United for Separation of Church and State, with headquarters in Washington DC, needs volunteer support in every community to ensure that all public schools are nonsectarian.

Drivers will feel useful volunteering for Meals on Wheels, assuring shut-ins of a daily hot meal and some cheery words. Or perhaps a local church group has meaning for you, though it's tough to tell whether it's the God part or the community aspect that does the heavy lifting here, according to a study on the science of happiness conducted in 2005 at the University of Illinois by psychologists Ed Diener and Martin Seligman. Both psychologists found, in their research, that service benefits the giver perhaps more than the receiver.

I've yet to hear of a political campaign office that turned down any offer of free assistance for their candidate, providing their candidate is also your candidate of choice. The atmosphere is loaded with enthusiasm bordering on antic and you'll be hugely welcomed by a new group of people. There's always an air of exquisite comicality that strikes me as downright theatrical among political zealots, which is good entertainment in itself.

Volunteerism can be far more than your gift of community service, it can be a learning pathway to place you in a better position for paid work in the future should you want or need it. You're also allowing yourself chances to meet new people who are as generous as you are with their time; wherever generosity exists you'll find solid friendships. For now, however, the idea is to use personal liberty as occasion to learn new skills and to join a greater community of stimulating new people who do things that make a positive difference. You can also see it as one way to take charge of your new single-again life.

2

Give Talent a Chance

If you've lost a loving companion of many years, certainly you're dealing with a legion of feelings; it's a lot to handle alone. Loss and loneliness are a mean combination. Yet I can imagine that it's also made you more appreciative of the very significant role of true partnership.

If you're alone now because of a divorce, it will likely sharpen your determination to make a better choice the next time around.

Either way, you're on your own for the first time in years, probably not on very sure ground. It's natural to feel lonely as you adjust to the reality of being single again after all your years of partnered life. But no one should be lonely or defenseless forever, and you don't have to be. It's not up to others to take away your loneliness, however. You must take charge of your own social life.

Try to think of someone whom you would call a successful widowed or divorced person. What makes him or her that way? Think also of other healthy-minded men and women who were at one time in the same position in which you now find yourself, and look closely at how they remodeled their lives to be much happier for it. Then think of those who wouldn't make the effort, and what do you see? Who are the smartest survivors?

Difficult as it may be to accept, it's your attitude toward change that will be key to improving your life. A positive attitude to make the most out of your life can save your life. I'm not talking about changing your personality or flaunting yourself publicly or doing anything in any way embarrassing, just a willingness to enter into new constructive situations that bring you pleasure with new experience.

My friend Mitzy loves to entertain, and the first summer after her husband died she treated herself to a very expensive week-long cooking course given by a French chef in a centuries-old chateau in the countryside near a charming French village. She was immersed in a totally different culture in a safe environment soaking up new ways to prepare foods and wines. Doing what she loved to do, she soon forgot her uneasiness at being on her own. One of the men who took the course with her in France came to Montreal last summer to see her again; it's not a romance, but it's a strong friendship based on common interests. Any travel agent can put you on the right track to this kind of cooking adventure in Mexico, Istanbul, Spain, Italy, Asia, wherever. All you have to have is a passport and a fat wallet.

What you presently have going for you is time. Time to call your own. Time that *is* your own to indulge your secret ambitions, to look at your creative side. Perhaps you've often thought you'd like to improve your photography skills, yet you lack technical knowledge. You can do it! With a small investment of cash for supplies and registration in a photography class, plus a steady mix of determination and self-discipline, you can do anything you want to do.

Where to start? The field's wide open and your choices are almost unlimited: workshops and classes in painting, dance, jewelry design, pottery, and sculpture are likely on offer at community colleges and public schools in your community. Fiction or nonfiction writing and theater workshops are other options, as are classes in gourmet ethnic cooking, hat design, department store window dressing, and magazine editing—the list is endless. There's nothing to stop you now; it's your turn to try your hand at whatever you've always been curious to see if you could do well.

Inexplicably, some people are just plain gifted, born that way. My son, Ross, I swear was born with a pencil in his hand—at least it felt like it when he was bumping around inside me for months jabbing sharp blows at my ribs! And way before he hit kindergarten he could draw a sleek car you knew was going too fast, or a man headed for a painful pratfall on a banana peel. It's a rarity to know instinctively how to draw expressively; most of us, however, have latent talent that needs schooling to shine through.

When time is your own you can concentrate on your creativity. Give it priority. Later on you may prefer working alone or working commercially, but the opening move is to get yourself back into the community in situations that motivate and connect you to a network of people with similar interests. Provocative people with fresh ideas are the ticket, because creative men and women are always attracted to one another.

Workshops are great places to improve your craft and to hear thoughtful critique from your peers. These classes are usually small, eight to ten people. You'll also find the same welcome reception in foreign film or journalism seminars, in a faux-finish painting workshop, and in screenwriters' workshops. If you sign up to study in a field that is of true interest to you, you will be perfectly at home and meet the kind of people with whom you have much in common. Often it's your avid interest in a subject, but not necessarily your expertise, that makes a bond with others.

No doubt there are various galleries in your city where photographers, sculptors, puppeteers, jewelers and glass blowers show their work. On a quiet afternoon's browse of one exhibit you might easily strike up conversation with a fascinating person who's enjoying the same work that's caught your own interest. Notice that I said person, not man or woman.

Remember this: almost every person has aunts and uncles, sisters and brothers, friends, sons or daughters, nieces and/or nephews. Through just one good person you can meet an entire company of new friends. Whenever you meet a new interesting person, you are pre-connecting with a wider band of people, all the time broadening your circle.

Gallery owners will gladly add your name to their invitation lists for opening night receptions if they know of your interest. Tell them you're attending courses. Or tell them you occasionally buy a painting. But even if you're neither a student nor a collector, your goal is to be around others who are creative or simply appreciate creative output.

Get out the yellow pages and call around to all the galleries you like best and ask to be put on their mailing lists for new shows.

Talk to people at these openings about the art on display; head straight to the person you feel might be the most richly innovative individual in the room. If you've mistakenly chosen a certifiable nut case, so what? Move on, there are others in the room.

But you could also get it absolutely right and meet someone with whom you have a lot in common, someone who likes doing the same things that you like doing. Perhaps it could lead to a lunch and a day of flea marketing or a theatre matinee. Man or woman, it doesn't matter, you're simply looking to extend your contacts with other creative people at this point.

Just going to gatherings and standing in a corner of the room isn't enough. Wishing that the perfect woman or man will single you out is plain dumb. When you're in a room filled with attractive people, circulate—look for someone standing alone, and go over and ask how he or she likes the artist's work. Get a conversation going; you are, after all, trying to get to know new people. To listen and learn about art and why a certain artist works in a certain medium or employs a certain technique is a life-long study for an art lover. Bring others into your circle with a smile or a comment such as, "Come and say hello to us."

Do your part to make the gathering a success and you will be invited back again and again to other openings by the different gallery owners. Each time you mix with art lovers, you will see more familiar faces, you'll greet and be greeted by name, and pretty soon you'll be recognized as one of this tight-knit group yourself.

3

How to Jump-start Your New Single-again Social Life

For my friend Luz, cooking is pure enjoyment. She's wildly enthused about foods and wines.

We met for lunch one rainy, cold October Saturday in Toronto's classic French restaurant "Le Bistro" on Queen Street. Inside the restaurant the low-ceilinged intimate atmosphere and delicious aroma of baking bread welcomed us. I was happy to be shot of my soggy blue tweed coat and more than happy to let Luz order a simple lunch for both of us. She's good at anything and everything to do with food.

In her lovely Cuban accent, she ordered bowls of green pea soup, thick slabs of rough country pate with tart crisp red apples, and ice-cold unsalted butter with fresh warm French bread. From an overhead breadbasket on a pulley we landed the bread to the table and polished off an entire loaf with the perfect potage aux pois.

The tables were spaced far enough apart to allow for quiet conversation. She told me she'd always felt perfectly comfortable around kitchens and good food, but she was exceedingly uncomfortable in the current dating climate. Jake, her beloved husband of thirty-one years, had died very suddenly of leukemia almost two years earlier when Luz was fifty-eight.

She was bursting to tell me her news. She told me she'd started a cooks' dining club. She'd been very selective in putting the group together, as she'd wanted to gather superb cooks who were also deeply interested in politics, art, literature, ecology, global news, science, and the idiocies of our legal system. She got what she wanted—an informed, compatible group of easy conversationalists, none of them smokers or joke-tellers, all excellent cooks in one or another specialty. She knew that a diverse, interesting group would last a long time.

What made it special was that every invited member had lost his or her mate of many years. Each member was alone again after death or divorce had ended a long basically reliable relationship with his or her partner. Three members of her group were divorced and five were widowed. She often mentioned Ron, one of the widowed men, and I just grinned. "Oh, you! Stop that!" She flicked her red linen napkin at me, but her face was flushed, and she was laughing like she had a wonderful secret; I never did get a straight answer out of her.

The last time I'd seen Luz, she was depressed and hurting. She hadn't said so, but it showed in her face and the way she spoke: her voice registered little interest in anything or anyone, including herself, and her shoulders sagged as if they were holding up a continent. That was then. She looked so different now—excited about her life, her cooking club, and her new friends. Luz had organized the cooks' club on her own because food was her comfort zone, and she'd brought other older singles into the area where she was at her best. Smart lady.

Of course, not all of us enjoy cooking as much as Luz and her friends. Perhaps you would rather eat than cook? You might consider forming a dining out club made up of single-again men and women who are game for trying new places to eat. Each week a different member searches out an inviting new restaurant, calls everyone with directions, and books the dinner reservations.

Groups like this work best in large cities where there are congeries of fine eating places that specialize in an infinite variety of cooking disciplines. It is also a good idea for each member to occasionally bring in a new member to change the group dynamic and prevent cronyism. If you want to hit the top restaurants, keep in mind that groups of eight persons tend to get loud and no one wants a table anywhere near a noisy group. Two smaller tables for four would solve the problem.

Books and writers may be your first interest; if so, you may enjoy a book discussion group. It takes no outlay of cash; it's simply a matter of inviting a couple of widowed or divorced friends who can suggest other men and women book lovers who are alone again and interested in the idea. The best groups never get too large; around twelve is a good number since not all will make it to each meeting. Also the best book clubs never advertise.

In preparation for the initial meeting, someone—probably you if you're the one forming the club—can choose a solid, well-written, compelling work of literature. Allow each person plenty of time to get the book read before the first meeting. Try to keep the group fairly evenly balanced between single men and women. Once you decide the kind of group you want to form, you can create an ongoing social situation quite naturally. It may begin as a private book club meeting at members' homes, but can at some point grow to encompass activities at booksellers' events or lectures. It may develop into a potluck lunch and book club. The members will come to know one another well over time, and strong relationships can form within the group.

Most public libraries sponsor oral readings on a regular basis, often with the author in attendance reading from his own work. The readings are terrifically popular. Book lovers are interested in the process of writing and publishing as well as in reading the product. Very often the reader will take questions from the floor. There are break periods at these events that allow time to have a few words with the speaker or with someone else who brought up an interesting idea in the discussion. This is a great breeding ground for new friendships between book lovers.

Another popular group activity is mall walking before shops open up for the day. You meet at a starting point and go from there. The larger enclosed malls open their concourses to early morning walkers in hopes that their window displays will excite buyer interest. If you exercise at a good stride regularly, you'll probably drop a little weight and pick up a new walking companion. Any mall store manager can give you the name of the operations director of the complex for information on time and place to join the walk. In the summer the area is air-conditioned and in winter it's heated. More importantly, the surface is not snowed on, rained on, or decorated with dogs' business cards.

Or you can organize your own walking tours for a group of single-again walkers to investigate a different section of your city each week. Some museums host historical walking tours in the older parts of their city. It's easy enough to find out how they work by calling the tour coordinator, and you can join their already formed group. However, the biggest advantage to forming your own club is you get to limit membership to widows, widowers, and divorced men and women. There's nothing wrong with married people; it's just that they're married. And you're not.

Another thing to keep in mind when you meet someone through a walking tour, or even walking your dog in the park, is to look for women or men in your own age range. A little younger is okay. A little older is okay, too, but big age gaps aren't wonderful if you're looking for an ongoing attachment.

In the middle years, wide age differences work, and they work well. At either end of the spectrum they don't. A thirty-five-year-old man with a ten-year-old girlfriend gets locked up. Good! Better he should be castrated. A seventy-five-year-old man with a fifty-year-old woman isn't thinking. It's one thing if a far-apart-in-age couple has had many good years together to grow into old age, but for *any* man (doesn't matter how young you feel) to start a new relationship at seventy-five with a woman twenty-five years younger is not smart. It sounds more as if you're looking for a nurse. It's bound to be a more comfortable situation if you choose a woman nearer your own age, one who remembers roller-skate keys and multiplication tables—a woman who's at least heard of Guy Lombardo. In fact that could be your opener: "My dog's name is Guy Lombardo. Remember him?"

A movie group is a favorite with film buffs. It can concentrate on a certain genre, such as foreign films or early black-and-white art films. You meet at the theater or at another location (for example, you may be able to view films at a local library), at a pre-decided time to see the movie, after which everyone goes out together for a drink to discuss story lines, actors, directors, special effects and production. Pretty soon new friendships are formed thanks to common interests. Start with a couple of single-again friends who will each invite another newly single man or woman friend—*not* one they themselves are interested in romantically—thus widening the web for everybody. If film is your favorite entertainment medium you're in good company.

What you are doing is planning activities to suit your own special interests and, in so doing, creating new possibilities for a broader social life instead of waiting for someone else to make the first move and then drag you along. Taking charge of your own life is what self-reliance is about. Autonomy doesn't mean you can't rely on others at times, but it *does* mean that you don't have to.

4

Shyness Is Not a Good Enough Reason

Extremely shy men and women will find being single again both desolate and scary. But loneliness is a killer. It sucks any joy straight out of your soul. Even if you are afraid, there are simple, comfortable steps you can take to meet new people.

Years earlier in life you met the one who turned out to be your future spouse at school, at a summer job, or at a university. Back then there were family reunions and church gatherings, and young people met and married friends of friends. Or perhaps once school was left behind there was travel to another country where you formed exciting new connections with traveling companions.

You met in the workplace, on a ski hill, in the Peace Corps, at Labor Union meetings, in the park, in drawing classes, at a CPR training session, at hairdressing school, at medical school, at political rallies, and at sports events. Perhaps you met through business or industry, at a conference, at a gym or a dance hall, on the assembly line, in teacher's college, at a rock concert, or in the armed forces. Each different situation brought with it the possibility of new acquaintances.

These easy grounds for interaction no longer exist in the same quantity later in life. But living alone, and staying home to read, write, do house and yard work, sit in front of a computer, watch TV, pursue a hobby in your own workspace, or baby-sit grandchildren is no way to allow for new friendships. These are all solitary pursuits. And anyone who lives alone behind closed doors is never going to find a new love.

You can be the most fabulous person in the universe, but without a solid plan of action to get back into circulation as a single-again person, who's ever going to know it?

Who would even know that Rita, a bright, funny, socially awkward, fifty-year-old divorced artist, wishes someone wonderful would arrive on her doorstep and fall in love with her and her watercolors? It just isn't going to happen, because no one knows she's available. She holes up in her studio and works long hours alone.

Delores is a painfully shy sixty-three year old esthetician who is crying (literally) for a new person to love. Her husband came back from Vietnam tragically addicted to drugs and died years later of an overdose at age sixty. By day she advises women on skin care, and in the evenings she reads romance novels; she imagines herself as the heroine who gets all the hugs, and she wonders if a face-lift would make it possible.

Both Rita and Delores need to look for a safe environment where they will meet with the same group once or twice a week: an excellent choice would be a series of classes in welding, a twelve-week course in computer repair or fly-fishing instruction. Each of these courses can and do accept women and men, but the enrollment will lean heavily to male participants; therefore, there's greater likelihood of them slowly becoming friends with an interesting man. Whereas a twelve-week course in hat making or jewelry design will attract mainly women, but shy guys who sign up for those particular courses have a good chance to get to know a lady classmate.

Jacob, a reclusive seventy-seven-year-old engineer, is longing for emotional attachment, but he hasn't told anyone because he's embarrassed about feeling lonely at his age. Throughout his entire married life he was the positive strength. He loved taking care of his wife and afforded them a wonderful life together. Now she's gone and he doesn't feel strong at all.

If you're shy, then it's probably more difficult for you to make the effort to meet new people. But shy is fine—it's okay to feel awkward.

The thing to remember when you meet a new person is that you want to see what you have in common. Shared interests and shared values are what you're looking for. When you find common ground and can say "me, too" or "I know exactly what you mean," you'll be more comfortable. But absolutely nothing is going to happen until you get out of your apartment or out of your house. Out of the house and involved in the community in a way that allows you to make new friends. And not just any friends—you have to frequent the kind of places where you will meet compatible people with whom you share interests and who you will get to see regularly. Since shyness doesn't make for dynamic first meetings, it's helpful to put yourself in situations where you will be among the same people on an ongoing basis.

When I was first divorced and blonde and living in Mexico (it doesn't get better than this, believe it—Mexican men will build a chapel for a blonde), I met a charming man in an art gallery. He was a concert pianist/composer attending an art gallery opening for his younger brother's paintings.

I was at the gallery because I'd bought a fabulous drawing done by Alejandro Colunga earlier in the week and was invited by the gallery owner to meet the artist at the reception. But it was the artist's brother, the music man, who completely bowled me over. Within weeks we discovered we both loved original art and opera and jazz, street parades, sassy kids and marching bands, Mexican history, old black-and-white films, and hot dogs with mayonnaise. We both loved to read novels and to write; he wrote music, and I liked to write stories. We shared a quirky sense of humor; it's easy to understand why that relationship lasted for years.

A shy, quiet woman I knew casually in my Spanish class became envious; she was curious as to how and where I'd met Bernardo. I told her. "Wow, I'm going to start hanging around art galleries," she decided on the spot. But it didn't get her anywhere, because she wasn't interested in art and had practically nothing in common with anyone who was. Her interest was spectator sports. When she started coaching girls' soccer, which she truly loved, her shyness disappeared. She met the single father of one of the girls, and they eventually married.

All of that happened umpteen years ago, but the protocol hasn't changed and the rules of conduct are the same now as they were then: *you meet the most compatible mates when you do the things you like to do best.*

You need to sit down and make a written list of those with whom you've been most comfortable throughout your life. Start with the boys and girls you chose as childhood playmates. Keep going with the list right through your choices of high school and university friends, business colleagues, single and married friends. The reason that you felt close to certain people, and not others, is because you shared common interests, true? There's your big clue.

A widowed friend of mine works part-time in a bookstore. She just turned fifty-six and is kind of timid. However, she says the bookstore is a perfect place to meet and talk with male customers: they constantly ask if she's read a certain book, and, if so, what she thought of it. She's an unslakeable reader, and thoughtful questions from customers erase her shyness; she's in her element talking about literature. She's also a raging Democrat and gets to hear a man's political views if he picks up a presidential biography or a book about a certain candidate's thoughts and theories. And, she added, if he makes a purchase she gets to see if he has platinum credit. When I joked that she sounded more like a closet Republican, I received a fierce scowl.

To meet a man or a woman who can be a potential love-interest you need to be, on a regular basis, in a place where you have a sense of agreement in speaking and working with people you respect and fully enjoy. Especially if you are shy, it may take you a while to work up enough courage to speak to someone who attracts you.

If you like taking pictures, a photography club that meets every Wednesday, for example, will give you repetitive exposure to other photo club members who want to improve their camera technique.

From a common interest, conversation springs naturally out of the activity at hand and your shyness is forgotten.

A choral group's regular practices would allow time to get to know another choir member who has your attention. Love of music is what brought each choir member to the group in the beginning, and that common bond all but eliminates difficulties in communication. The only tricky part is you probably have to have at least a passable singing voice, so this option is not for everybody.

Whatever activity or interest group you choose to join, involve yourself in practical ongoing situations where you can become properly acquainted with its other members. You can offer to help edit the group's newsletter, pick up a member who doesn't have transportation to the meetings, make coffee, or stack chairs at the end of a work session.

Are you well above average intelligence? There's a place for you in Mensa, a worldwide high-IQ club, after you pass a qualifying exam. However, having a high IQ doesn't equate necessarily with people who always put their brains to good use. A members' mailing list can, and does include not only some brilliant minds, but anti-social misfits and some clever caught-criminals serving time. I had a German friend in Mensa who left irritating messages in classical Latin on his answering machine for callers to decipher. You can imagine how many people got back to him. A quick call to Mensa will give you current meeting times and locations in your area. Their web site has several entertaining intelligence tests you can try.

If you're concerned about homeless people living on the streets in your city, or you want to help raise funds for AIDS research, the appropriate groups are eager to have you join them. You will have the privilege to meet selfless people who are willing to do their part to make the world a better place; you'll find good people here.

Perhaps you're passionate about rescuing greyhounds from the racetrack and placing them in good homes, or working with an environmental group to clean up our beaches and lakes. The importance of a watchdog coalition to preserve the separation of church and state might have your attention. Or you feel a compelling need to help eliminate the shocking degree of illiteracy in the country. You're vitally interested in putting together a literary magazine for young people to slow down the loss of teenage readers who put increasing demands on electronics to do their thinking. Just name your dream. There are groups of activists who share your feelings and value what you value, and it's among people who give gladly of themselves for the betterment of the community where you'll find the highest potential for strong friendship. There's no room for shyness among passionate people. You'll meet incredible men and women for lasting friendships and, sometimes, romance.

I know a married couple that met when they separately joined Habitat for Humanity. They were concerned about the growing numbers of families unable to find decent affordable housing, and each of them was sufficiently moved to try to help in some way. They're both quite shy, but they blossomed as they helped to build a house together. Today, side-by-side, they continue to support Habitat's building projects. The most generous-minded men and women are drawn to projects like Habitat.

TIME Magazine investigated the science of happiness in a special mind and body issue (Jan. 17, 2005). The research done by various psychologists found that being fully engaged in meaningful activity topped the list as one of the greatest sources of true happiness. And when you're truly happy other people want to be near you; your surge of energy sets off a positive response in others that invites personal relationships.

Worldwide Volunteer Vacations is a pay-your-own-way group that sends volunteers to teach in different countries. It's not necessary to actually be a teacher. Your job can be to sit and talk with Italian schoolchildren who don't have the opportunity to use the English they are learning in an Italian classroom setting. Italian kids want to know what kids their own age in North America like to do, what they wear, if they have part-time jobs, and how much freedom they have. They also want to pick up American slang expressions. You will work long hours: eight per day with the children and possibly Saturday mornings with the resident Italian school staff. You'll be housed with an Italian family. In the evenings, you'll be shown the sights by your host family and teachers and by new friends.

Where you don't meet anyone is staying at home behind closed doors waiting for someone to come and rescue you. Feeling sorry and helpless doesn't work. Loneliness is solvable, but the responsibility rests with you alone. Shyness is not a good enough reason for isolation; it's an excuse. Besides, shyness is kind of an insult to other nice people; it's as if you cannot trust another person with your fears. Some trust is needed here.

The first step is to find a group activity that fully captures your interest. Or find soul-satisfying paid or unpaid work—part-time, full-time, whatever suits your situation. Look in the newspaper. Get out the phone book. Start making appointments for interviews in places where you can work alongside men and women who share your interests and concerns. The reference desk of your local library is a good place to inquire about different interest groups. Or you might locate a comprehensive list through your local community center or the chamber of commerce or the Unitarian Church or a Reform synagogue—institutions that are all well known for their involvement with the community at large.

Just do it! Let yourself have fun with other people and guess what? They're going to love a not-so-shy-after-all *you*!

5

A Man Talks to a Woman on the Move

Whether it's a day trip to the casinos, a tour of artists' studios, or a longer vacation, you'll meet more people if you take that trip alone.

Friends who own a ski lodge tell me they won't accept reservations for a dozen girls on holiday together because no boy staying at the lodge wants to approach a huge group of girls to single out one from the crowd.

It is no different when you add forty or fifty more years; a lone man, even with added maturity and confidence, will still feel too awkward to come near several women traveling together. He won't. Here is some advice given to me years ago from my brother, Al: "I can't tell you how unapproachable a group of older women looks, whether on a plane, a train, a bus, or in a restaurant or hotel lobby. I wouldn't have the nerve to speak to just one woman in a group at a swimming pool, a lecture, or the track. You can be pretty sure that if you go on a trip with a group of women, you'll come home as a group without having met anyone new.

"If you have the courage to go alone on a Victorian Houses bus tour, for instance, you have a much better chance to meet and spend time with a new man who may well turn out to star in your future happiness. You already know that you have common interests, or you wouldn't have chosen the same outing. Another good day trip to do alone is a vineyard tour if you live near wineries. Between a small orientation talk given by a knowledgeable grower or winery staff member, a conducted walk through the vineyards, a tour of the cellars, and a few wine-tastings, it's pretty easy to chat with fellow visitors and some of the staff."

Sounds like good advice from my brother, who wasn't at all shy, yet wasn't interested in attempting to single out any one female from the herd, either. No matter how self-confident, no man willingly stands in the way of possible rejection.

When you travel alone, travel light. Avoid worries about hanging around for checked or missing luggage, or lugging suitcases through concourses. My great friend Jody Allan, a noted Florida-based artist, doesn't blink an eye about taking off alone on a bus in Mexico for five days with nothing but a canvas tote bag holding cash and one credit card, a toothbrush, an extra shirt, a sweater, a book, and her camera. Period. She talks with everybody when she's photographing. Like Jody, I had done a similar three-day bus trip from Toronto, Ontario to Naples, Florida, luggageless; I had my passport, money and toiletries in a shoulder bag, and I wore four pairs of panties, which I discarded one by one from the skin out in the various bus terminal washrooms along the route south. Obviously you can't lose luggage when you have none. At stopovers I had coffee with fellow travelers; after each bus stop there was a fast shuffle of a few seats to continue talking or to get a card game going.

Not everyone has the opportunity to travel, but the same general idea applies to other activities that allow the possibility, should you want it, of conversational contact. One painless way is to sit at a diner lunch counter instead of in a separate booth with your nose in a book. You're much more approachable at an open counter. In addition, if you put something weird, such as a snow-globe, in front of you on the counter, it can whet the curiosity of the woman or man seated beside you. And suddenly, you're talking.

If you live near the shore, try walking alone on the beach. Most beach walkers tend to get out good and early, before it gets too hot or crowded with sunbathers and the picnic crowd. Smile as you walk, and say good morning to everyone. Keep moving along, but not at such a breakneck pace that you appear unsociable to someone who might want to walk along with you or pick up beautiful shells and enjoy the morning together.

I'm not meaning to imply that everything you do has to be done alone in order for you to meet new people. However, if you go every single place with the same friend, and you laugh and chat cozily together, obviously having a great time in each other's company, it's apparent this is a closed circle and no outsider is particularly welcome. It's lovely to have warm friendships, but if you truly want to find a new woman or man partner in your life, it's smart to allow time for some adventures on your own.

A single ticket to a concert series (a series, not a single performance), can place you next to another single-ticket holder. This happens. But you don't have to leave it to chance, you can request to be seated next to a single male or female ticket holder when you purchase your seat; no one will know. Series tickets are usually sold in pairs, so it makes sense that two people holding one ticket each will be seated beside each other.

I know a married couple that met this very way. They were both divorced. She was a cello player in her late fifties, and he was an Irish tenor in his sixties. Neither of them was a professional musician; they were just two music lovers. At first it was a few remarks as they took their seats. Then it was "hello" and "how are you" at the next concert and a drink together at intermission. As they were leaving the auditorium after the final concert of the five-part series, he asked her to have dinner with him, and as she nodded agreement with an all-knowing cosmic smile, he asked, "what's so amusing?"

"It's my guess you waited till the last concert to invite me out so that if the date didn't go well, we wouldn't have to run into one another again."

His mouth widened into a huge grin. "I adore clever women."

Now he's still grinning at that clever woman—across their breakfast table.

6

A Widow Makes It on Her Own

Tillie married at twenty and was widowed at sixty-four.

She had never managed her own finances, she'd stopped driving a car as soon as her son Bruce was born, and in all forty-four years of married life, she hadn't worked outside her home. Her husband liked to be in charge. When he died she was hopelessly dependent, and fully expected her forty-year old son to take over running her life. Her son, however, had other plans, and, not incidentally, so did his wife.

Bruce encouraged Tillie to take driving lessons. On the day she got her license, he arrived with flowers to celebrate his mother's move toward independence. Tillie was truly excited with her achievement. She planned to have her husband's sedate black Cadillac repainted pale rose. Bruce bit his lip, but he hugged her hard. "Congratulations, Mom. What's next—a job? Get to be a big tycoon so you can keep me in style?" He was teasing, but Tillie really liked his idea of a job.

She arranged for an interview in a bookstore, but without computer skills, she was unemployable. She wasn't able to order books online from a wholesaler or search for a book title on the net.

"I would have been so good for that store. I've been a big reader all my life, and I could have helped customers find good books," Tillie told Bruce later that evening on the phone. "Here I thought I was going to tell you I'd landed a job for one or two days a week, but no go."

Tillie put a little edge of snob in her voice, imitating the bookseller, "Sorry, my dear, but in nearly all retail shops, apart from antique dealers or one-of-a-kind craft studios, you really need to be familiar with computerized inventories and ordering practices. To put it flatly, you have no marketable skills."

"She really put me off when she called me 'her dear'! And then when I applied for work at the kitchen boutique," she went on," same response: without computer skills we can't use you. I was truly stunned! I was one of their best customers. Do you know how many times I showed them how to use a new piece of cooking equipment I brought back from Portugal or South America? Or brought them a wonderful garlic press I picked up in France or a set of perfect copper cookie cutters that I'd got through a catalog I felt they might want to stock in their store? And what's more, they did add them to their inventory, and made money from my suggestions. Damn them."

"Kind of discouraging for you, Mom, but you have to understand what they're saying, even though you know more about cooking and cooking gadgets than practically any one of their clients. In today's retail world, computer literacy is a must. Listen, you've heard the phrase 'if you can't lick them, join them?'"

"Tell me."

"Just get a laptop computer and take a course in how to use it at a vocational school."

And she did. The computer classes were a total failure. I mean utterly *total*. Tillie simply couldn't master the computer. She hated both the machine and the instructor, who went too fast with his explanations. But her determination to succeed in business had surfaced and wasn't about to fade away.

Her confidence level surprised Bruce; he'd never seen this side of his mother's personality, and he was proud of her. "You know, Mom," he said to her on the phone, "you don't need computer skills if you work for yourself. Years ago you said that some day you'd start a cooking school. Remember when you taught me how to make spaghetti sauce?

Now all my friends ask me to make it when they come for supper. You could still do it, you know—open a cooking school."

Slowly Tillie replaced the receiver on the hook and, with more daring than she'd ever shown in her entire sixty-four years, decided to follow her long-time fantasy to have a small cooking school. Sure she was nervous about her ability to make it work, but she didn't lack courage. Fear plus action is the recipe she chose to follow.

She knew perfectly well that the majority of men her own age and older do not cook. Old men eat. A novel idea was brewing in Tillie's mind, and she felt a surge of eager impatience to put her plan into action; her liveliness made her very attractive.

She rented space in a church hall to teach cooking classes to single-again men *only*. That was her brain wave. No female students at all. Only widowers, and divorced older men coming out of long-time marriages.

She advertised in the church bulletin and in the local newspaper. Her enthusiasm for her cooking school was catchy, and the classes filled up fast for her short three-day courses. Easily half of her student enrollment was prompted by exasperated daughters and daughters-in-law either worried or fed up with a single-again father or father-in-law, and even one grandfather who couldn't or wouldn't make his own meals.

Along about her fifth week of teaching, one of her repeat students, a widower in his late sixties, invited her to Sunday brunch at The Ritz. Tillie, who hadn't dated in forty odd years, was giddy as a schoolgirl.

Except for a new dress, new shoes, new handbag, manicure, pedicure, facial, haircut, and color—which ought to take care of the cumulative profits for her next six months in business—she's all set and couldn't be happier with her life. At the age of sixty-five, Tillie now has a career for the first time in her life, a career that comes with its own captive audience of eligible men.

Tillie's no dummy!

If Tillie's idea catches your imagination, there's nothing to stop you from doing the same thing. Most women who have kept house for years know how to cook. Also, quite a few older widows or divorcees on fixed incomes need to earn extra money.

A lot of older men don't know beans about cooking, but would be willing to pay for classes if it meant they could learn how to make something more interesting than fried eggs and bacon.

If you arrange to hold classes at a synagogue or church, there'll be a rental charge for the kitchen, but it's better to pay the fee than it is to have strangers in your own home, especially now that you're alone. You can ask another widow or divorcee to help with the classes, particularly if she's a lot of fun and has a specialty in an area of food preparation other than your own. It allows for "insider talk" in your classroom demonstrations to have a second cook—you've likely seen the success of this format on TV cooking shows.

Start with a short three-day course of classes on a Monday, Wednesday, and Friday of the same week, with three different meal plans as daytime lessons for beginners. Simple supper menus are the ticket, such as meat loaf or shepherd's pie. Egg dishes and ham croquettes are good options as well. Fill out the menus with a variety of side salads and various rice, potato, or pasta concoctions. And any guy can learn to master the art of a butterscotch sundae or a fruit cobbler. You'll have lots of ideas.

With each weekly course you'll want to vary your menu plans, because some men will wish to continue with more lessons. In addition, you need to investigate new dishes to cook to maintain your own freshness as a teacher.

You'll probably want to kitchen-test the recipes at home to see how long they take to make from scratch. As you go along, your menus can always be refined to fit your budget as well as your schedule. You'll have some arithmetic to do to compute your food costs, the rent for the church kitchen, plus the cost of an assistant. The figure you arrive at will dictate how many students you need to enroll to cover costs and make a profit. Tuition should be affordable yet still be worth your time and energy. Usually classes of this kind last for three or four hours, and you can look forward to some hilarious afternoons.

It's easier if you and your assistant do all the cooking while your students watch and take notes and give you lots of good-natured banter from the bench. Beforehand the men can help with the hands-on scut work of peeling, chopping, mixing, and stirring—and probably a fair amount of mess-making—so add extra-large blue denim aprons and hefty sponges to your shopping list! Working together in a class is an ideal way to have fun and make good friends.

When the meal is ready, students and cooks sit down together and eat "the lesson." Wine makes it festive. However, you'll have to check with the church secretary to see if you can serve wine in their kitchen. Could you call it "communion?" It is a church, after all, but really this isn't the kind of fib that sends you to hell.

On the matter of cleaning up the kitchen, you'll likely get some resistance, so make sure it's understood from the get-go that dirty pots, pans, and dishes are part of the curriculum. Let your students know that any man who cooks and cleans up his own chaos will definitely rate high with the ladies.

Men who cook are at a premium, and men who cook well are often better cooks than women, but, most of all, men who cook are plenty cute.

7

Three New Beginnings

Go ahead and yell your head off at the unfairness of being alone again, totally unprepared to handle everything by yourself. It won't do you a bit of good to scream, "Unfair! Why me?" Mostly it's a big waste of time. Instead you might choose to take positive steps to conquer your fears because fear of being alone is mostly what it's about.

It's natural to be frightened and under-educated in your new situation. It's an enormous change in your life to be alone again after so many years as half of a solid team.

A proven way to gain self-confidence and the respect of others is to find work that interests you and to do it with all-out enthusiasm. It can be volunteer work. It can be part or full-time paid work. It can be at-home or on-line income-producing work that you invent, but perhaps at-home work isn't your best present choice because an important aspect of work for you is to reconnect with the community.

Above all, don't focus on the fact that you've haven't held a job in a long time (perhaps, never) or that you have absolutely no current job skills. Or that you're too old or too fat or your neck is crepey or you don't have a wardrobe of power suits. It will only discourage you further and if you fall into that trap you're one dead duck.

Here are the tales of three resourceful people who were left alone abruptly. Each of them needed additional income, which, in its self, motivates fast action if it doesn't flatten a person outright. Not one of them had the credentials to interest a potential employer in today's business climate. Instead, they each took responsible action by creating jobs for themselves and, in so doing, discovered romance along the way.

Noah is fifty-six. He started out as a fashion illustrator in the ad-art department for a national magazine. He married young. However, their only child was born retarded when his wife, Ethel, was forty. The event changed the course of his career. He quit the magazine for freelance work in order to share the constant care needed for little Jeffery. They moved to a roomy, neglected farmhouse near a popular skiing area.

"I'll never forgive myself or forgive you for producing a retarded child." There was steel in Ethel's voice.

"She can't mean that. She'll be just fine once she stops feeling guilty for having a mentally handicapped kid," Noah's sister insisted.

"I don't even see him as handicapped or retarded. Jeffery's a sweetheart; why can't she see that? Why would anyone feel guilty about having a beautiful, precious child? I'm going to teach him a lot of things and make his life into something any boy would envy. And you don't know Ethel as I do. She's stubborn, and once she decides something, there'll be no change of heart."

"Give her time, Noah." And he did, still Ethel remained distant and cold.

Noah spent all his free time with Jeff. He taught him how to pick up his toys and look after his room and make his bed. Together they planted vegetables and flowers. Jeff loved watering the plants and soaking his father with the hose and jumping up and down with glee when Noah ran to grab the hose and turn it back on Jeff, hooting with laughter, "I'll get you for this, you rotten kid!"

When his son was older, Noah showed Jeff how to make simple meals and do careful house repairs. Jeff was more of a slow student than mentally deficient, and in the patient, loving climate that Noah created, he blossomed.

When Ethel was killed in a three-car collision on an icy winter night, all Jeff said was, "I wish I missed her more, Dad." He was twelve years old.

"Me too, son. I wish I missed her, too."

Both Jeff and Noah found life a good deal more pleasant without Ethel's disapproval, and together they decided to open the farmhouse to paying guests; Noah needed to create a livelihood for Jeff's future. They turned the five-bedroom house into a bed-and-breakfast. It was a small enough operation for Jeff to cope with easily; they never had more than three rooms rented overnight.

Noah taught his son simple accounting, and Jeff turned out to be a whiz at numbers. When Noah got a computer, Jeff proved to have an uncanny aptitude for the machine, which is not unusual for slow learners with keen interest in a certain subject.

With a popular ski area nearby, "Jeffery's Inn" had full bookings all winter. A year into the successful business venture, along came Katie, who stopped over at the inn on her way to a dog breeder's show in Boulder City.

Katie was in her late fifties, wonderfully warm and homey. She told Jeff and Noah splendid funny stories at supper about breeding Border Collie puppies and how she kept the entire first litter for herself because she couldn't bear to part with even one of them. And how her then-husband hated dog hairs on the furniture and finally left her for a stainless apartment and a Decree Absolute. "Whew, what a relief!" Jeff shouted and giggled at Katie.

On her way back from the breeder's show, Katie booked a room at the inn for a whole week. She had two new dogs with her. One was a stud, perfect for breeding purposes, and the other, a gift from Katie, was an eight-week-old puppy that drank Jeff's potato soup, peed on his shoe, and then settled snugly into his new owner's arms and fell asleep instantly with his cold little nose tucked under Jeff's sweater. Jeff was in heaven.

That did it. Noah wasn't letting Katie get away from him. Nor did she want to go anywhere. She married him in the spring of that year at the farmhouse with Jeff as best man and five beautifully groomed Border Collies sitting at attention. Katie was the woman Noah loved and had always wanted. Katie was the mother Jeff loved and had always needed.

- *Some vocational schools list short courses on operating a bed-and-breakfast or longer courses in hotel and motel administration in a typical year's calendar. Bed-and-breakfast operations do well in cities as well as in rural areas. They are especially popular in locations known for their tourist attractions. Comprehensive books on the subject are available at your public library and at your favorite bookstore. There's also a wonderful program called Innkeeper For A Day, which you can access through the Internet. It offers an amazing opportunity for anyone contemplating opening a bed-and-breakfast to have a trial hands-on experience at an actual country inn.*

I first met **Beth** at an aerobics class a year after her husband dropped dead during an important tennis match at Wimbledon. "Oh, don't feel sorry for him," she said quickly when she saw sympathy in my eyes, "he wasn't even one of the players on the court. He was in the bleachers drinking lemon squash heavily sluiced with gin, a cute habit he'd been perfecting for years."

Beth is sixty-two years old, casually stylish, and good fun to be around. Her married children live in various places across the country. She started her own unusual gift basket business after taking an evening class on that subject through an adult education program at a local high school shortly after Freddy went to his reward in a haze of gin.

She goes around to large office buildings six weeks before Christmas with flyers advertising "Lingerie Gift Baskets for a Lady in Your Life." Men flock around Beth to use her shopping service; she solves their biggest headaches every year.

The most popular items are sleek satin nightgowns with spaghetti straps, filmy peignoirs, and high-heeled mules with marabou trim. Perfumes, lacy teddies, handcuffs, garter belts, and fishnet stockings are other hot items.

"A huge percentage of men think peek-a-boo black lingerie is the ultimate choice regardless of the lady's personality, age, shape or coloring. I mean it—the end of the world could be at hand, but a man will still hang onto his fantasies, no matter how ridiculous. It's a bit like a little boy giving his mother a baseball mitt for her birthday.

"Often a male shopper will want to include packages of condoms in the gift basket. It's a good idea that I encourage," Beth said. "One time I was out with Olivia, my thirteen-year-old granddaughter, and she wanted to fall right through the floor in the drugstore when I asked for eight dozen French condoms in pastel colors and polka dots. She's been leery about shopping with me ever since."

Beth shops strictly within limits of an agreed-upon budget for a particular client. She wraps the gorgeous lingerie in heavily embossed silver papers with shimmering silver ribbons and arranges them on a sea of shredded cellophane in a sterling basket topped with huge organza bows. The entire silver extravaganza is tented in crisp clear plastic, finished with fabulously baroque crimson silk hibiscus flowers. It's her signature wrap.

She's been doing her exclusive Christmas lingerie baskets for four years. They're hellishly expensive. Her business is growing so rapidly that next year she'll hire an assistant and start filling the orders weeks earlier.

When Beth married Freddy he'd had rather a lot of money, but years of pursuing the party life of drinking and frittering had seriously depleted his capital. Beth's gift basket business affords her a much better life than she would have had had she relied solely on what was left of Freddy's thin estate.

"And now the good news," Beth added with a charming smile. "A former girlfriend of an executive client of mine was downright insulted by one of my gift baskets that he sent her. And she decided to return 'his damned tacky present,' as she called it, and stop seeing him altogether. The idiot woman didn't have a teaspoon of wit! Now Cecil invites me to dinners in fabulous restaurants around town, and I adore going places with him. He's wonderful company, and I think we're falling for each other."

- *Adult education programs are offered typically in high school classrooms during the school year on weeknights. Course schedules are generally made available in public libraries at the start of a school year. If you don't find a course on creating gift baskets, I suggest enrolling in a short business course to learn the rudiments of purchase and sales and to understand the basics of accounting and profit margins. Then go around to the finest specialty food shops and examine the gift basket displays carefully. Fruits, nuts, wines, caviars, and chutneys may indeed be totally different from the items you want to handle, but unless you master simple business procedures as well as the art of exquisite presentation you cannot hope to succeed in a luxury gift basket business.*

Jessie is seventy-five years old. I think the woman is amazing. When she was seventy-three, she underwent a mastectomy followed by the standard therapies, during which time her husband walked out on her. To be fair, he wasn't a total louse—they hadn't been a strong couple for a long time, and she hadn't been the greatest wife.

Jessie had worked for an insurance company until she was fifty, so she had a small pension plus her social security benefits. What she needed was part-time work and more money to live on. However, twenty-five years after her retirement, her job skills didn't mean twit in the current market. Employers, in general, are nervous about hiring anyone over sixty-five. It's something to do with insurance coverage, I'm told. Wal-Mart, happily, is an exception to the rule, and so are many grocery chain stores such as Publix. They both, as well, hire handicapped persons who are able to do the work.

In the "classifieds" Jessie found an ad from a publishing house looking for freelance copy editors. Her age wasn't a problem, and neither were her qualifications, after she wrote a completely bogus letter of glowing recommendation from an out-of-state publisher hoping it wouldn't be checked. It wasn't. When Jessie's back was against the wall, she did what she did to survive without having to apply for an assisted-living allowance. I'm not advocating anyone telling lies exactly, but it did work. Sometimes you do what you have to do.

Her attention to detail was excellent and she got all the copy work she wanted. The cash was good. The one drawback was she lived a near solitary existence working alone at home with no interaction with other people. Then along came a new manuscript from the publisher for her to check; it dealt with tracing missing persons, and the more she read the more fascinated she became—she knew she wanted to work in that field.

When you're adventuresome at a young age, the cockiness doesn't disappear in later years. Jessie was a maverick as a girl, it seemed she still was. However she knew her limits physically and didn't see herself as a private investigator chasing sweaty, knife-wielding men through darkened back alleys. She was a little eccentric, but she wasn't totally crazy. Where she could see herself was as an assistant in a PI's office researching leads by telephone and on the Internet and following the paper trail that any person alive leaves in his or her wake.

Jessie got on the phone to more than a dozen private investigators before she found one that would listen to her. Her gutsy manner impressed an investigator in a one-man operation, and damned if he didn't hire her on a trial basis. She argued that as a copy editor she was meticulous in the detailed work of checking book-length manuscripts to see that nouns agreed with verbs and to make certain that the publisher received clean copy with correct facts, grammar, punctuation and spelling. She convinced the man that she was an excellent researcher.

The investigator began bragging about Jessie and the swell job she was doing for him, and somehow it caught the attention of a television journalist who was putting together a segment on employed and employable men and women over normal retirement age. The show highlighted Jessie's story, and the station got a lot of congratulatory mail on the piece. One e.mail sent by a retired cop to invite Jessie for lunch sounded promising, and she asked her employer to check the man out. The report on Sam, a retired widower of three years, was A-OK all the way.

Jessie and Sam met for lunch at a neighborhood diner that caters mainly to cops. She loved it. "Hey, sleuth!" Sam said and stuck out his hand to give hers a hefty Irish shake.

"If you're interested in me, that's okay. If you're interested in my job, you can't have it," she shot back, and they both started to laugh.

Immediately they were in cahoots. They both talked a mile a minute, and they had each other's full attention throughout the meal.

Unbeknownst to either Jessie or Sam, Jessie's own PI boss sat at another booth double-checking that everything was aboveboard. He couldn't be too careful with his favorite employee, after all. As he watched them having fun together, he had an uneasy suspicion that there'd be some changes in his office staff soon.

- *The Yellow Pages of your phone directory lists schools for private investigators. To have that particular training under your belt would be solid evidence that you can be a useful behind-the-scenes assistant. You can also check with your local library for books on tracing missing persons; anyone interest in the process of detection will find the material galvanizing.*

    The Complete Idiot's Guide to Private Investigating, by Steven Kerry Brown, a former Special Agent for the FBI, is an excellent book that is available at your bookseller's.

8

Shake Up Your Chances for Romance

SITUATION #1: You're a man who loves big band music, yet you never invite a woman to go dancing because you feel ridiculously awkward on the dance floor.

SUGGESTION #1: This is going to be fun to fix! Sign up for some dance lessons, and your attractiveness will triple—guaranteed. Your effort alone is worth an A+ from any woman. It's not necessary to be competition with the likes of Gene Kelly or Fred Astaire; they danced in the rain and on a ceiling for heaven's sake. You don't have to go that far! It's enough to be willing to learn a few dance steps and how to relax on the dance floor and stay off your partner's feet. Holding a woman in your arms while dancing smoothly to your favorite music is a very good move that you can count on doing again and often.

SITUATION #2: You're a woman who travels every winter with the same woman friend to a sunny climate where English is spoken. Each winter vacation is an echo of the one before. You're dying to go to Portugal, to France, to Viet Nam, to Tonga, but it's all so foreign.

SUGGESTION #2: Why? Why settle for unromantic trips? You are a single adult woman, free as a bird to go anywhere you can afford at any time of the year. How about taking that vacation alone where you're certain to be more approachable? Go ahead—I dare you!

Young girls travel in pairs or in groups. They need one another because they're not very sophisticated or sure of themselves, but grown women often have greater adventures alone.

Once you choose an exotic location, an intensive language course to correspond with your destination is a must to kick-start your trip. Supplement the classes with foreign language tapes and DVDs that you can borrow from your public library; you need to simplify your travels by learning key phrases for directions to the post office, bus stop, washroom, telephone, taxi stand, or sidewalk café. "Where can I purchase ten yards of red velvet?" (a phrase actually taken from an old "Beginning French" Berlitz curriculum) is *not* a key phrase, since you certainly won't be sewing living room curtains in your charming French pension on the Left Bank. Another swell item you can purchase from Radio Shack-type stores is a battery-operated hand-held gadget on which you can write an English word or phrase and it gives you the French translation on the spot. Conversions into other languages are also available.

In the travel section at any bookseller you'll find helpful guidebooks for the country of your choice with excellent current information on places to stay, and on restaurants and shops as well as not-to-be-missed points of interest. You could meet the love of your life when you do something so different from your ordinary routine, because the excitement will show in your face and in your manner. That kind of attitude is magnetic; people around you will react very positively and want to be near you.

SITUATION #3: You're a woman who's worn her hair the same way for the past fifteen years—a bit dated maybe? Mostly you wear dark skirts with a white blouse and a solid colored cardigan sweater. Pearl studs in your ears. Your makeup has been unaltered for years as well; I'm guessing tawny beige foundation with coral lipstick?

SUGGESTION #3: You're begging for a change. Call a top modeling agency, tell them you're in need of a change, and ask if they'd be good enough to give you the names of two or three top hair stylists where you'd get a great haircut. Phone around and get their prices, then take yourself off to the most expensive stylist you can afford (take out a bank loan if necessary). Because he's so sought after, as well as wildly expensive, do not tell him what you want for a style. He's the expert; let him give you his expert advice on cut and color. Yes, color! Highlights, whatever. Then call the Estee Lauder cosmetic counter in your city's top department store and ask for an appointment with their best esthetician to help you up-date your skin-care products and makeup. Be prepared to take notes because that person will be well trained by the Lauder group. The service is free. You don't have to buy everything he or she suggests, but get the basics to give yourself a fresh, natural look. As for your clothes, what you've been wearing sounds safe and easy, but it also sounds as if you're in a boring rut. The better dress shops have sales staff who are up on the latest and best in fashion, or you can ask a man or woman friend, who has that great "put together" style we all envy, to help you find a new look. When your look is updated, you'll be feeling so much more confident that others, too, will see you in a brand new light. In their book *Closing the Deal*, for women who want to go from single miss to wedded bliss, authors Daniel Rosenberg and Richard Kirshenbaum advise women to market themselves if they hope to interest commitment-phobic men. Its reference to women in advertising terminology may strike you as a bit crude, but you know precisely what is meant. And they are correct: it's practical because it works.

SITUATION #4: You're a creaky male with stiff joints, especially in the morning when you first get out of bed. Your condition makes you feel at least a hundred. It's a shame for you to feel so uncomfortable when you can do something to lessen your discomfort.

SUGGESTION #4: Yoga classes will loosen you up and have you more agile within weeks. If you can't manage all the weird stretches or bends, just do what you can. In time, if you stick to the program, it will benefit you enormously. And the odds are in your favor to meet some good-looking limber women, because more single woman than men participate in yoga programs. This is a winning solution!

SITUATION #5: You're an interesting woman who sincerely longs to meet a new man for friendship and perhaps romance. All the men in your circle of friends are men you've known for years; you're all used to one another, and no sparks are flying in any direction.

SUGGESTION #5: Sign up for a course in television repair, or car repair—very few women, make that almost no women, sign up for these courses, so you'll have your pick of all the men taking the same course. It's useful to know how your car works, even if you still plan to call AAA or CAA when you get into trouble on the highway. For the odd time when your car won't start or it's making disgusting sounds, it's nice to be able to make a simple adjustment or, at least, be prepared to describe the problem properly to the mechanic when you call the garage. And the mechanic who answers your call and fixes your car may be a prize, too, so you can ask him out if you want. It's not up to the guys to do all the asking anymore.

SITUATION #6: You're alone again after years of being half of a married team, and you feel ungrounded. Unanchored. You think of friends from your past who you've not seen or heard from in years. Regrettably, over time, you've lost touch with them.

SUGGESTION #6: You can start with your high school and/or university alumni association to ask about reunion dates and current addresses of some of your old classmates. You can call one or two old friends whose addresses or phone numbers you do still have, and ask them if they know the whereabouts of other old friends. Classmates.com is a useful Internet site that may offer possible leads. The Internet also provides people searches that you can access through your own desktop computer; men will probably be easier to locate than women who often go by their husband's surname. The telephone directory can be another helpful tool if relatives of your friends still live in the area. Little by little, one name will lead to another and your list will lengthen and reach into other states and provinces and even other countries. Perhaps there was one special girlfriend or boyfriend from your past that you've thought of often over the years who you'd love to see again. I recommend an excellent book by Nancy Kalish called *Lost and Found Lovers*. It contains facts and fantasies of rekindled romance.

She says it can be so amazing to learn your lost love has thought a lot about you, too, over the years. And who knows? Maybe she or he is also alone again.

Plan a vacation to travel across the country looking up old friends. Send a postcard beforehand (less threatening than a letter), telling of your "old friends tour". Take any old photos you have, along with news of local people they used to know. Pre-book motels or bed and breakfasts everywhere you plan to visit, and invite everyone you contact out for dinner on your tab. Then move on to the next place. At each stop you'll pick up additional names and addresses of lost friends to include on your route. If you go by car you're more flexible and can stay longer than originally planned in any one place if it suits. Without question this will be a trip to remember; who knows what can come of it? And some of your old friends will likely want to visit you next summer.

SITUATION #7: You've lived in the same house since shortly after you were married thirty years ago. Some furniture you bought together as a couple, some you inherited and placed exactly where it sits to this day all these years later. In fact the interior of your house has looked the same way for as long as you can remember.

SUGGESTION #7: You're single again and it's beyond time for an overhaul; you're way overdue. Don't even mention that it would be disloyal to your dead wife or husband to make drastic changes! Loyalty has nothing to do with painting a wall or upholstering a sofa.

For starters you need to freshen your living room, bedroom, and bathroom walls, ceilings, and doorframes with a change of color or colors. Even if you quite like the present color, change it. A line of paints, by Debbie Travis, groups compatible colors to depict certain moods: dramatic, romantic, soothing. They are beautiful colors. After you've done painting the initial areas, you can go crazy on the rest of the house and the exterior, too, if you have the cash. But mainly what's important is to get going. Give your home a jolt to wake it up. Move the furniture around; a popular trend in furniture placement is feng shui, which is thought to invite harmony into your living space. There are plenty of feng shui books available, or an interior designer can present you with a complete plan for paint colors, furniture suggestions, and fabric choices for upholstery. Just don't pick a fascist designer who insists on making all your decisions for you. Will decorating your house change your life? No, but it will change your outlook. You can expect to feel energized and livelier in your new surroundings, and you'll want to have friends over for dinner or to play board games.

SITUATION #8: You're a woman who's been on her own again for a few years now, and, in all that time you haven't met anyone romantically special to you. You dine out casually with women friends on a regular basis.

SUGGESTION #8: When you travel to another city, you eat in the best hotel dining rooms by yourself. Why do you find it's easier in another city? Try dining out alone at top-rate hotels in your own city. Try different hotels, places you don't ordinarily frequent. Make a reservation for yourself at a visible table next to the dance floor or floorshow. Get your hair done, dress your prettiest, order a glass of champagne once you've been seated, and, above all, relax. This can be entertaining! Look around the room, and if you spot a nice-looking man having dinner by himself, give him a friendly smile and lift your shoulders in a mock salute as if to say, "We're both in the same boat." Don't be surprised if he sends a drink with his business card to your table. Hey, a little flirtation is fun; it makes you feel alive and recognized. And by giving you his card it puts the ball in your court to respond if you wish.

If it's an option, choose the buffet menu; you can fix yourself a small plate when an interesting lone diner is at the buffet table. Make sure it's a small plate in case you get nowhere with your first prospect and want to go back to the buffet again without splitting the seams of your dress when another fine solitary man is helping himself to the lobster bisque.

SITUATION #9: You're alone for lunch in a café or diner. You usually sit in a booth with a book.

SUGGESTION #9: I've mentioned this before, but it bears repeating. Head for a seat at the counter with an unoccupied stool on either side of you, or sit beside a person who catches your eye. Do not stick your nose in a book; lay the book or, better still, some colorful travel brochures on the counter beside your water glass; it gives your neighbor an opener to talk to you. A big brass and silver French horn on the counter is good, too—huge and questionable, but difficult to ignore.

SITUATION #10: You say, "I'm over fifty, actually quite a bit over fifty, and I'm not having any luck finding a new mate."

SUGGESTION #10: In a lively book by Rachel Greenwald called *Find a Husband After 35* (forget the title—it still applies for older people), she says the first thing to get rid of is your coffee maker. Instead get out of your home and drink coffee alone at Starbuck's or Tim Horton's every day. She calls it breaking out of your bubble. Her proactive approach to dating is based on what she learned at Harvard Business School to solve business problems. Get her book immediately to learn her five top tips for singles looking for a mate. Ms. Greenwald outlines a strategic plan, much like a plan you would use to accomplish any other goal in life, such as finding a new job. She recognizes that dating can be intimidating at any age. Though it may seem a tremendous challenge, a few positive changes in your life can make finding that special someone to love far easier than you ever imagined. There's no time like now to go to your bookstore and find this workable book. Who knows? You may find your perfect someone right there in the bookshop in the same section looking for the same book.

9

Take the "A" Train

How long has it been since you traveled by train at ground level instead of in a plane where the only sense of motion you feel is possibly a little turbulence? Where you can actually see and feel your movement through the changing scenery instead of wondering what part of the nation is far below as you fly above the clouds totally out of sight of land? Where you actually have the visual adventure of traveling to a new place, rather than just leaving one airport to arrive at another?

Car trips don't count, because they're usually fraught with frustrations of consulting maps, calculating mileage, watching out for speed traps, stopping for gas, waiting in line to use grungy washrooms, staving off hunger with disgusting fast food, and trying to find a motel en route. Mostly a car trip is exhausting and it's what's called "getting there;" it is not a vacation.

A trip by rail across Canada can take you from the older settled east coast at Halifax through the Maritime Provinces and exotic French Quebec, to the exciting and culturally rich city of Toronto. You'll ride past the wheat fields and grain towers of the Prairie Provinces, perhaps with a stopover to attend the annual Calgary Stampede. Then on through the magnificent peaks of the Rockies and breathtaking Lake Louise to the stunning younger westernmost Canadian city of Vancouver. I'm talking about the trip itself being the true vacation. If you have a computer, all the information you need to help you choose a travel package is on the Internet. Google "train travel/Canada."

Crossing an entire country by Viarail in Canada will likely take seventeen days or, depending on what you choose as your package of extras and side trips, you might decide to do twelve days from Toronto to Vancouver or five days from Calgary to Vancouver through the Canadian Rockies. There are similar length trips by Amtrak in the United States. All the rail excursions offer captivating side trips.

Luxury train travel—with bubble-domed observation cars and restful sleeping accommodations, gourmet meals, plushy rotating seats to watch the passing scenery in the bar/club car, with seasonable stops to experience well-chosen points of interest—is not inexpensive. In fact it's probably a-once-in-a-lifetime, memorable, deep-hole-in-the-budget grand tour where time loses meaning in a relaxed, leisurely atmosphere.

There's a lovely feeling of lush sensuality in having five-course evening meals in the softly lit dining car with snowy linens and silver cutlery, crystal goblets, and tasseled menus. Pretty dresses for the ladies and dinner jackets for the men add a touch of formality to dining on a first-class train; it is akin to the ceremony of cruise ship meals at sea. Even during the day, if you're curling up with an interesting book in the club car or enjoying tea and conversation with another passenger, casual clothing means cashmere sweaters and fine wool slacks for both men and women. Leave your jeans and sweats in a bottom drawer back home.

It's interesting to observe the same tour passengers as the days go by, to get to know some of them better than others. Even if you're a shy person, a week on a train is ample time to become close to a fellow traveler who interests you. Now we get to the part about traveling alone. For some travelers this takes courage, especially the first time you go on a trip by yourself, but if you give it a try, you'll see for yourself that it's a real eye-opener; you'll meet and get to know people you would not have met if you were traveling with a companion.

Traveling by luxury train or by cruise ship allows plenty of time to see if someone who catches your eye has a positive outlook and interesting things to talk about, as well as time to investigate any interests you might have in common. Both by sea and by train you are a member of a community of travelers in the roomy yet enclosed space of a moving hotel. You'll find out who is an attentive, thought-provoking dinner partner and how he or she treats waiters and other service people; you'll see if he or she eats with a closed or open mouth. In the club car, you'll learn who drinks moderately or too heavily, who reads what kinds of books, who's fun to play cards with, who's pleasantly self-confident, who fidgets or talks incessant nonsense, who's clever, and who is the liveliest company on a stopover in one of the cities along the way. Eight days of close proximity certainly holds the possibility of changing the very course of your life.

You'll come back a changed person because of your exposure to a rather outdated method of transportation, a novel way of socializing, and perhaps even a special attachment to one person in particular who is destined to be the love of your life.

Other shorter trips of two days (without stopovers) can start in Calgary, Alberta, and take you through the majestic Canadian Rockies to Vancouver, British Columbia, for much less money, yet still a thrilling trip. There is also the Whistler Mountaineer run: three hours by rail from Vancouver through spectacular terrain that hugs the Pacific coast, with unrestricted views of the 8,787-foot domed peak of Mount Garibaldi and the impressive cascade of Shannon Falls from the bubbletop observation car to reach the sophisticated mountain village of Whistler.

Internationally, there are trips to the Copper Canyon on the Al Pacifico Railroad that runs through the state of Chihuahua, Mexico; the Copper Canyon is breathtaking in grandeur and, to some, more spectacular than the Grand Canyon in the United States. To learn more about this never-to-be-forgotten trip, go on the Internet and "Google" Copper Canyon, Chihuahua, Mexico, and it will bring up glorious color photographs, testimonials and press releases, info on airfares and gateways, plus a request form to fill out for a free brochure on the various canyon tours and accommodations.

Dartmouth University alumni continuing education and travel programs and Harvard University Alumni tours also have programs available, albeit not by rail. You can sail to the United Kingdom on the *Queen Elizabeth 2* with a professor of Shakespearean studies and onboard classic Shakespearean films, plays, and lectures followed by trips to Stratford-on-Avon and the Globe Theatre in England. Other Dartmouth University alumni educational tours will take you, along with a Greek scholar, through the Mediterranean by ship on a journey back in time to better understand the past island life of ancient Greece. Yet another offering on their program is "Hiking the Inca Trail: Machu Pichu": immerse yourself in myth, legend, and history of the Incas. You can learn more about all the marvelous tours to exotic places with Harvard or Dartmouth approved professors as your guides by bringing up Dartmouth Alumni Continuing Education and Travel on the Internet. Search the site or send for a brochure of upcoming events.

If you're in excellent health (they tell me fifty is the new thirty), and don't have the finances to travel at lofty prices, you could cruise the world and get paid for it! Cruise lines are seeking at-sea administrative and entertainment staff to service cruise ship guests. Perhaps you have teaching experience in art, writing, tap-dancing, computer skills, photography, backgammon, bridge, or theatre arts. There are many slots to fill to keep high-paying customers on world voyages amused at sea. You can fill out a job application online at http://www.cruiseshipjob.net, the biggest cruise ship staff hiring body in the United States.

You could cruise the world and get paid for it! Can you think of a better place to find romance? Shipboard romances happen all the time at every age, and if you're lucky enough to be working on the ship, you will meet everybody—staff and guests alike.

10

Fresh Places to Look for New Friends

A man on the scent at the perfume counter

You're in a department store when you spot a very nice-looking woman you wish you could meet. She stops at the perfume counter to try the spray testers and talk to the salesperson.

Over you go. Stand close enough to be seen, but far enough apart not to infringe on their conversation or make her nervous. At some point the sales assistant will turn to you and say, "I'll be with you when I'm free."

"I'll be happy to wait. I need a gift for my sister's birthday, and I'm going to need some help." Smile at the lady customer (the one you think you'd like to meet), and tell her, "My late wife (or my former wife) used to say that women usually have a favorite scent. If I don't know it, I'm sunk. Is that true?"

This is a perfect situation. Women love a man who's unafraid to admit he needs a woman's help. This will result in conversation. Keep it light. Smile a lot, but don't get flirty. So even if this woman you wanted to meet turns out to have a very much alive-and-kicking (a swift kick if he knew what you were up to) husband at home, tell her you enjoyed talking with her and give her your card. She may have a friend who's a widow or a divorcee she thinks would be a good match for you. Perhaps she'll include you on a future dinner party list. And, so far, you haven't embarrassed yourself or her by being flirtatious or dumb.

If you never hear from her, you still have your sister's birthday present. If you don't have a sister, it's far too late and quite impossible for your parents to provide you with one.

A puppy helps a man find a suitable lady

A man with a dog is good. A kind of goofy puppy with floppy ears and paws he hasn't quite grown into is best—the kind that has women saying, "Oooh, you're so adorable!" Meaning the dog, of course.

If you don't have a pup, borrow one, or discuss a walk-for-a-fee service with a veterinarian in your city. You could also offer to walk a working friend's pet to a pleasant park every afternoon where you hope to catch the attention of a charming woman who you feel wants to catch your attention as well.

Try different times of day at the park until you see a woman who looks approachable, and to whom you could introduce your puppy.

A lady goes shopping in the men's department

Men's Harris Tweed sports jackets and small-size men's dress shirts look very chic on women. And where do you expect to find them? How about in the men's department of a large store such as Macy's or Saks Fifth Avenue? Actually, your nearest and largest department store is where you start.

You're going to try on men's jackets in the men's department and ask a good-looking male shopper, "So, what do you think: does this jacket seem too big for me? I like it, but I don't want to look like I'm all shoulders." Your opener gives him specific questions to answer.

Let's say he says, "Turn around. Well, I think maybe you need a smaller size, you're not a big woman." That's positive. He's giving you consideration. He sees you have a small figure.

Now it's your turn to move the conversation a little further ahead. You can say, "I wear a lot of black in the winter, and this gray and black herringbone will be useful. You sure it doesn't look too mannish?" If he's enjoying you and wants to keep this dialogue going to get to know you more, there's probably only one thing he *can* say, "Oh, no! You could never look like a man!" Next he gives you his card. The guy's a pushover—almost too easy. But you get the idea.

Knowing the age and type of man you'd like to meet will help you pick the appropriate time and the store where you think he would shop for clothing. For example, you won't find an elderly Brooke's Brothers type at The Gap after school.

A retired man probably shops in the daytime, before or after lunch. A single middle-aged man who is working downtown will shop on his lunch hour. A married businessman or a man with a girlfriend will shop with his woman in the evening or on a Saturday.

You can have a bit of flirty fun shopping in men's stores at any age and, from what an adventuresome neighbor tells me, you won't be disappointed. She always meets men this way.

Get a haircut where the men go

You do not need to go to a hairdresser for a blunt cut. You can go to a barber. You sit in the row of black Naugahyde and chrome chairs with all the other guys and wait your turn. Choose a chair near the end of the line beside a man who looks like he'll be fun to talk to, with an empty chair on the other side of you for a second man should the first one speak only Czech, which, unless you happen to be Czechoslovakian, wouldn't get you anywhere. Park your coat and bag in the vacant chair until a good prospect comes along, and then you can move your things to give him space.

You only get to do this kind of scouting every three months unless you plan on going to the barber's every day and ending up bald inside a week.

Go to a popular barbershop with only one or two barbers on duty between ten and eleven o'clock. The line will move slowly, giving you more time to chat with the man beside you. At that hour of the morning, he's either retired or the president of something, since he's not rushing off to his office. You look at him and smile, "I've been going to the same barber in Chicago for years, but I've moved here recently and I want to find another man to do my hair. Which one cuts your hair? It looks good," you tell him.

"I have Julius cut my hair." Then he'll ask, "Where in Chicago? My daughter lives there with her husband. Since my wife died, I go to Chicago twice a year for a few days at a time."

Just look at how much information he's given you to work with! He's interested in your hometown. He's told you he has a married daughter and that his wife is dead. That's very good. Yours is the next move.

"I also like the idea of seeing my son for a short visit every four or five months," you say. "Much easier on everyone than one long visit each year. Never did believe in living my kid's lives." And the conversation goes back and forth from there till he asks, "How about taking our new haircuts out for a coffee when we're through here?"

This goes under the heading of a pick-up, but no one's in trouble. No addresses or last names have been exchanged. If all goes well over coffee, and he's introduced himself properly, you can tell him that you really enjoyed his company and give him your phone number. If you've had a good time with him, and sensed he was having fun too, then you can count on hearing from him again.

When he calls, if you absolutely cannot have lunch with him on the day he suggests because of a long-waited-for dental appointment, tell him, "It's so nice to hear from you. But listen, I've been waiting for my appointment with Dr. Christie for a month. Can we meet the following day instead? Or perhaps you have a better idea?" By naming a specific alternate date, instead of "why don't you call me again sometime," it lets him understand that you really do want to see him.

Browse the movie rental outlets

Friday evenings you'll find Blockbusters, and other movie rental stores, especially crowded with male and female browsers searching the racks for their weekend viewing entertainment. If a certain someone in the store interests you and you wish you knew him or her, then make it happen. Say hi, ask if he or she has seen either of the DVDs you're holding in your hand, and if the answer is yes, ask whether the movie was exciting, dramatic, romantic, or what? That's enough of a starter to a conversation on your part; if the other person wants to continue talking, she or he will.

The more up-scale the neighborhood, the more well-heeled the store's clientele, so look like a winner when you go browsing, but don't, for heaven's sake, plan to go home to watch movies with someone you met five minutes earlier, even if you feel there's interest on both sides. How nutsy would *that* be? Instead, just write your first name and phone number on a piece of paper—no address or other information is necessary—and you will or you won't get a call at some point, which makes for a bit of fun wondering at the outcome.

11

Meeting In Person After Meeting Online

By now we've all heard about someone who feels a strong attachment to a person she or he corresponds with on the Internet. Or we've read about it or seen it featured on a talk show. This tale is about Ben, an electrical engineer whose wife died two years ago. He hasn't dated; he's alone most evenings, and he spends hours on his computer since he discovered online chat rooms.

He's excited to meet a special electronic friend in person: in this case, Anna, a woman he's come to know through a rapid exchange of revealing messages on a daily basis for the past six weeks. It seems boldness has power in the chat room, and Anna has become the focus of his thinking. The two have arranged to get together in her city; Ben already has his air ticket.

Talk show hosts would be six programs short each season if they didn't have guests who met in this fashion. And they all say the same thing: there is marked intensity to a relationship that starts on the Internet because of the speed of interaction and the strong protected conversational aspect of the correspondence. It's totally private—there's a notable and refreshing lack of interference from other people's opinions or remarks, and the distractions of business, children, and household duties are virtually nonexistent. There's a teasing quality to an online exchange, where you give little bits of yourself away each time you're on line together, but never the whole story. Since the person you "chat" with doesn't actually know you, has never seen you, and doesn't see your face when you're typing in a response to a question or posing a question of your own, it can bring out the cheap and charming in you. It can make you wittier and more daring, some would say reckless, than you are normally.

Most people who get involved on the Internet use an online handle rather than their real name (e.g., Wannawrite or The Fourth Tenor). It is safe practice to stick with the mystery until you can comfortably give out your true identity.

The computer, itself such a sterile piece of technology, doesn't count as a third party, therefore you can say things that you probably wouldn't say in six months of Sundays if you were together in the same room. It's human nature to present yourself ideally or, at least, as you think the other person wants to imagine you, and in this forum, you feel free to slingshot normal caution into the wind and just relax and revel in your own audacity. Now add to the mix the potent thrust of imagination and ego and you have enticing intrigue, especially if your real life at the particular time holds little or no excitement.

Ben got so carried away with Anna, with whom he spent upwards of two hours a night, he'd already decided she was the one he wanted to be with for the rest of his life. Keep in mind that while he is an intelligent, creative man, he was also a very lonely man at that point in his life and, even though they hadn't actually said hello face to face, they'd spoken by phone numerous occasions for hours at a time.

If you are presently involved with someone from a distant city whom you've met in a chat room or through one of the many dating sites on the Internet, you have to think carefully if you make plans to meet together in person. In the weeks or months that you've been "speaking" with each other, you've no doubt discovered common ground; let's say you're both interested in independent films and filmmakers. For sometime you've been dying to go to Sundance Film Festival, but during the past few years your wife was too ill to travel and you didn't particularly want to go alone. Now that she's gone and you're single again, the film festival seems an ideal way for two film buffs to meet.

The idea to meet an online friend for the first time at an event is good because the focus shifts to the event rather than highlighting two nervous personalities. You can still have a pleasant time with your new friend because of your common interests, even if you decide that true romance isn't likely.

You can get all the details squared away (separate hotels, or at least separate hotel rooms, and separate financial responsibility), before your travel plans are finalized; this will remove any dithers about possible expectations for both parties. It will also look after any guilty feeling you might have should you not want anything further to do with the person you'd agreed to meet. Intelligent advance planning will remove the hazards.

The two of you can also discuss in advance your thoughts about intimacy on this visit; it will make you both less edgy. There's all the time in the world to advance a relationship at a later date if you both decide it's what you want. If, however, one of you was expecting to shatter the commandments on the spot, then the effort to spend time together may be considered useless, and that tells you he or she is more concerned with ego than concerned about the new friendship. Therefore as soon as there's talk about a weekend visit, before either of you buys a plane ticket or makes hotel reservations and arranges free time, you must be up front about your expectations. Don't wait until you meet at the airport to have this discussion.

There's another serious pitfall. As soon as you make an actual date to meet in person, you can psych yourself up to expect that the person you are about to meet will turn out to be a dope who couldn't get anyone to like him or her unless the background information, interests, and values were all falsified.

Do you ever do that? Do you ever decide a worst-case scenario so you won't be disappointed? Try not to pre-decide the outcome of the first meeting. That kind of second-guessing can all but eliminate the possibility of any positive growth into the kind of relationship you truly want.

Instead, when you meet, try to put your new friend at ease by being relaxed, and don't try to impress with cleverness or winning ways. In other words, give the person a chance. It's enough to realize it's bound to be a goose bump moment when you first meet. He or she's going to be nervous, probably awkward, likely to say a few dumb things—just like you. And remember, whomever you're about to meet traveled a distance to meet you. And that person put him, or her self in a position where the result could hurt or disappoint or feel wonderful, so the desire to like you and to want to be liked by you is already in place.

Having said all that, the very best thing you can do for yourself, for your new friend, or for a fledgling relationship is to slow down and keep your balance.

If you live in the same city, it's so much easier to be casual about a first get-together for a drink in a popular bar at five o'clock. Make it spontaneous with a suggestion to meet that same day or evening and thus avoid the added pressure of high expectations. By keeping it simple, you'll feel more at ease. The person you are to meet will have your cell phone number only, not your directory-listed phone number, because it's not a big deal to change a cell number if you find that you don't want to pursue the relationship and want to avoid future calls. Leave your car at home and take a cab to meet your date to avoid having to walk to your car in a parking garage.

Or you might want to arrange to meet for lunch or an early supper—a popular cafe is good—but certainly not in either of your homes. Never give out your home address. Let a couple of friends know that you plan to meet someone who you've never actually seen, but with whom you've been corresponding for a while. Pick friends whose opinion you value highly, and ask if they would agree to have a meal in the same restaurant at another table and come over at some point to say hello. This gives you the chance to introduce your new friend to your old friends, perhaps invite them to join you briefly for a drink. You might feel these safeguards sound kind of juvenile, but it's always best to err on the side of caution. And if your date sees this "coincidence" as a set up, so what? He also sees that you're smart.

Quite often when a person is lonely, that very loneliness can affect judgment. After all, meeting a stranger when you already have a preconceived notion of what that person is about can, and likely does, place you in a vulnerable position. As a woman, you may have given off a few signals you wished you could have taken back five minutes after you high-heeled your way into a candid area.

A suitable person is an amazing find, a person who welcomes your attention as much as you welcome hers or his. An unsuitable person in your life takes up a lot of time. It's not better than nothing—it *is* nothing as far as you're concerned. What you want is to meet a companion who is right for you; if it doesn't work out this time, there can be other times with other people where it will work, so don't give up. Keep looking.

Going back to Ben and Anna, last I heard, they had a fantastic first meeting, and their plans are to continue to see one another as much as possible over the next year to see if this relationship is a lasting one for them. They both have very high hopes.

12

When You've Been Alone Too Long

It's been nearly seven years since your wonderful man died, and you're long past the status of *new widow*, yet in all those years you haven't met one man you can see as your new life partner. In fact you've become a kind of single fixture in a crowd of solid couples. Your friends probably feel you aren't looking for another mate, because you never mentioned that you'd appreciate their help to meet suitable new men; perhaps they think you're quite content on your own, if they think about your single state at all. How many dinner parties have you been to where your host evens up the numbers by inviting the same old perennial bachelor who has no curiosity whatever about women?

The best way to correct your situation, if indeed you want it to change, is to look after the details yourself. If you're not meeting people who interest you romantically, you need to get proactive and bump your social life into high gear by hosting a different kind of supper party in your own home.

How about asking all your single and single-again friends, men and women, to a potluck supper where the entry fee to the party is one casserole and one relative or platonic friend of the opposite sex? A single woman probably has a divorced brother, a widowed cousin, a single-again brother-in-law or her newly single nephew. A single male friend will have an unmarried female cousin, a widowed sister-in-law, or a divorced aunt. That way, everyone at the party gets to meet all the new possible interests without feeling that their own "date" is acting badly by flirting with one of their friends. You obviously don't care if your date/brother showers attention on one of your women friends who's caught his eye; he's not a womanizer, he's just your brother.

Some of your friends, no doubt, know attractive unattached friends or business colleagues of the opposite sex, in whom they have absolutely no interest romantically, who would love to join in the fun. What I like best about this idea is that you already know and trust your friends, therefore it's highly unlikely you'd have to worry about their choice of guests.

This is the kind of potluck supper party that has ongoing appeal and merits repeat performances as often as you like. It costs virtually nothing, as each guest brings his own food and drink. In addition, it's a party that maintains an even man-woman ratio, which adds to its charm.

If you and your friends like the idea of this kind of get together, you can vote to turn it into a regular monthly event and thus form your own singles club, encouraging different guests to join in.

If you're a guy, you can bring devilled eggs and invite a really funny divorced woman you know who volunteers at the library. Or maybe you're a lady and will bring chicken salad sandwiches and Jerry, a sweet, charming widower who lives on your street who you happen to know is very much wanting and hoping to meet a lovely woman to treat like a goddess.

13

A Great Quiz for Both Men and Women (to test your derring-do)

A certain amount of risk-taking is a valuable asset to a single-again person. Let's see how you measure up! There is no pass or fail; it will just make life simpler for you if you're willing to take a few chances to do things differently than you have in the past—mostly because there are so many things in your once-again single life that *are* going to be different. It's exhilarating to stretch beyond your comfort zone, because without some sense of adventure, it's hard to grow as a person.

True or False? (find a pen and write down your answers)

I like tough challenges.

I like to push beyond governing rules and make my own decisions.

I find societal restraints completely uninteresting.

I'm uncomfortable with people who can't choose, won't decide.

I'm suspicious of people-pleasers and false politeness.

I adore being in love.

I avoid people who say they're bored. Ditto with jealous people.

I form opinions quickly and enjoy having my opinions questioned.

I read a variety of books to satisfy a variety of interests.

I buy exotic vegetables and fruits at the supermarket. At times I haven't a clue what to do with them, so I spray them with white high-gloss acrylic paint to use as a centerpiece for a dinner party.

I have a terrific attention span for anything that grabs my interest.

I have the attention span of a gnat for moody or dependent people.

I admire originality and novel thinking.

I'm curious about how people think and their patterns of thinking.

I want a painted hot pink piano with purple polka dots in my kitchen.

I like to solve problems.

I'm fascinated with psychics and seers.

I want to go to Borneo and travel in foreign countries where I don't know the language.

I'd rather work freelance than work for a salary.

I'd be a good getaway driver for a bank robber.

Every day I wake up knowing something wonderful is going to happen.

If you had less than ten *trues,* see it as a wake-up call. How about signing up for banjo lessons? Or a course in bee keeping? Or lessons to master the art of engraving? You might take up line dancing, learn to yodel, take a helicopter ride over Niagara Falls, or read biographies of adventuresome men and women who went after their dreams. Tap-dancing is good, belly dancing is better, learning how to use a stripper's pole might be the best.

Zero in on Problems that Need Fixing: Part Two

14

Let's Get a Few Problems Out Of the Way

Here's the situation: You're single again for the first time in thirty-eight years, and you are very lonely. Recently an interesting man you met through friends at your golf club has been paying attention to you, yet you feel curiously uncomfortable with a brand-new person who finds some of your ways tiresome, or even irritating. So you're a little bossy. Big deal. Imagine the nerve of this new guy! It's been years since any man questioned your conduct. Is he the one who's a control freak, or could he be right about your bossiness?

It's always a choice to change or not to change a disagreeable habit. However, I think if you picked up this book, you did so because you wanted to see changes.

To change can be an enormous challenge.

Are you willing to take a personal inventory and keep all the best, most wonderful parts—the keen intelligence and charming personality traits—and toss-out, alter, or correct the annoying parts, the unattractive habits you slipped into during your former partnership? It's slack, almost too easy to get into conspicuously bad habits married to the same forgiving person for years and years. You're certainly not alone here; long-time familiarity in any relationship often cuts good manners to the quick. For sure it can be a joyride if you take up the challenge to drop the artless behavior and end up a happier person who's a whole lot easier for everyone else to enjoy.

Bad habits accumulated during the course of a previous partnership stubbornly prevent a surviving spouse from enjoying a full life with a new mate. It becomes almost impossible to put together a new relationship when there's old rubbish in the way. So take a deep breath and let's get to work. This isn't the time to resist.

The nagging wife in the car:

A bossy wife who delivers a stream of driving instructions from the passenger seat of the family car is annoying to be sure. But when she becomes a widow and continues to treat her friends or a new romantic interest to the same kind of directives that she issued to her husband for years, she's plainly insufferable.

Did you give unasked-for instructions to your husband when he was driving? Take your pick from the following list:

For heaven's sake, get in the left-hand lane.

Omigawd! You just missed a parking space.

Slow down, you damned fool—you're going to get us killed!

Don't drive so close to that car in front!

The list could go on and on and on and on and on. Did you never figure out how your husband got anywhere when he was in the car by himself without your irritating directions?

This is a joke I heard from my friend Emilie: A highway patrol officer pulls a car over and says to the man driving, "Did you know that your wife fell out of your car about ten miles back?"

"Oh, thank God, officer," said the driver, "I thought I was going deaf."

If you're on the lookout for a new partner in life, think about this—would you like to have *you* as a passenger when you're at the wheel?

The husband as mainlining critic:

Did you criticize your former wife for being frivolous with money or for the way she kept her checkbook? Were you on her back about her slap-dash housekeeping or the way she dressed or cooked? Did you disapprove of her friends? Did you dismiss her ideas as unimportant?

If you had helped her set up a budget and complimented her efforts to handle money, would it have been more effective? What would have happened if you'd pitched in with the housework and the cooking? Or told her how pretty she looked in her yellow sundress? Or spent time to get to know her friends? And credited her thoughts?

With a new love, your life can be much warmer and infinitely more satisfying if you give her complete loving support from the beginning. Start off the right way and keep it up.

Life can be so wonderful when a couple works together to help one another reap the rewards of returned affection. Certainly it beats picking away at your partner and being destructive. Being quick to criticize is a lousy habit, but hurtful habits can be broken when the desire is there for positive change. First off, figure out why you do it: are you modeling your behavior on a graceless example from your childhood? Serious conversation with a professional therapist about the practice of criticizing can be interesting and offer a lot of insight.

The picky wife as correction officer:

Did you pick lint off your former husband's lapel in public? Straighten his tie? Inspect his suit shoulders in front of others for dandruff? Make disparaging remarks about his hopeless grooming habits? Did you ever actually help him with his appearance? Compliment him on his haircut or choice of slacks or color of his sweater? Or did you simply call attention to less-than-perfect details?

Now that you're on your own again and starting to see other men, would you love it if your dinner date inspected your blouse in a restaurant for gravy spots? Or leaned toward you with napkin in hand (let's hope he doesn't spit on it first) to wipe lipstick from the side of your mouth?

Clearing up the clutter:

Over the course of your married life, how were you in the clutter department? Were the closets crammed with clothes, half of them either out of season, or things that didn't, and probably hadn't, fit anyone in the house for ages? Now that you're on your own again how about getting rid of some of the stuff? It's amazing how satisfying it can be to open a closet door and actually see what you're looking for.

It's surprising how your thinking clears up when you're free of mess in your home.

First you sort. This is essential. Sorting by category is one option: separate piles for skirts, pants, jackets, coats, shirts, and so on. Then there are shoes, boots, hats, and purses as separate categories, therefore separate piles. Or you can sort by seasons: winter clothes in one pile, summer things in another. Another method is by activities: clothes for gardening, fishing, tennis, or skiing.

You'll end up with loose clothing sorted in heaps all over your bed and draped over a couple of chairs, several piles on the floor, and some clothing hanging on the shower curtain rod.

Each pile will have things in it that you no longer want to keep; these articles of clothing get folded and put into large plastic garbage bags to take to shelters or Goodwill outlets. Broken, torn, ripped, and stained belongings get thrown out. Don't fool yourself that you'll fix damaged items because chances are, you won't. So far you haven't.

Rarely worn items such as evening dresses or dinner jackets, sequined purses, strappy satin shoes, bow ties, and cummerbunds can find homes in roomy plastic caddies that tuck neatly under a bed or in the basement; the see-through caddies are available in all Wal-Marts, KMarts, and other similar stores in various sizes.

Next you wash the walls of the closet, the shelves, and the closet floor before one single thing gets back inside it. Work on only one closet at a time, or it won't be just tightly jammed closets you're dealing with; the whole house will be one mammoth sea of clutter, the exact opposite of what you're trying your best to eliminate.

Are you in trouble here? If it's too overwhelming, a trusted friend or family member or even a professional closet organizer will help you keep up with the process. If you tackle it alone, sometimes heaps of memories impede or stop the project. It's nice to have someone to laugh with and share stories.

As you put each thing back in the closet, it's the ideal time to exchange all the give-away wire hangers from the dry cleaners for heavy plastic uniformly colored hangers for all your lightweight clothing. And use fat, padded hangers for your jackets and coats, dresses, best blouses, and silk shirts. Buy lots of sturdy pants and skirt hangers from the dollar store.

Smug. Positively smug. That's how you're going to feel when you're done. Oh, so what—another rotten habit.

Watch the applause meter, guys:

It's true there are fewer single-again older men than there are older widows and divorcees. Consequently these same women celebrate when an attractive man is unattached and available, and especially so when the man is witty, well read, and owns a decent looking suit. The invitations from single-again women keep such a man in a social whirl.

He appreciates the women who invite him into their lives, and he gladly reciprocates with phone calls, flowers, notes, and invitations to restaurant dinners and at-home parties. He understands a mutual exchange of privileges. In other words the man has class.

Another man who finds himself alone again after many years of marriage cannot use the "My wife used to look after all that" excuse, meaning the thank-you notes, phone calls, and return-invitations. He truly needs to develop his own responsible social skills in a hurry. Or he can revel in his present popularity for as long as it lasts, because it probably won't continue unless he catches on to the fact that there is, after all, an entrance price to any dance.

Never on time:

What you're telling people by always being late for an appointment or never being ready when someone comes to pick you up is, "you don't rate with me." You're saying, "you're not important enough for me to value your time."

This is probably the furthest thing from the thinking of someone who's chronically late, but lateness clearly affects friendships and partnerships in a bad way. Often, the very person who forces others to wait is impatient and annoyed with anyone who might keep him or her waiting even ten minutes.

Habitual lateness creates a lot of unnecessary resentments, and if it's your problem, then whatever reason makes you do it should be addressed if you're truly interested in being fair to your friends and family. This is a biggie needing immediate attention, and also one of the simplest things to fix. It's so common that most top psychologists probably have the cure for it on speed-dial.

15

Solitude Has Its Advantages.

To lose a life partner is devastating, but it's not the end of your life. You weren't the one who died. Your wife left. Or your husband died. Or your long-time partner died. You, on the other hand, are very much in the land of the living, and ultimately you are the only person who can help yourself. It's all about looking at your situation differently.

At the present time when you have a miserable head cold, you can splutter wetly and cough out loud in bed without having to smother yourself in your pillow so you don't make disturbing noises. You can turn on the light at three o'clock in the morning, go to the kitchen and get a liverwurst and pickled beet sandwich, and then watch reruns of Belgian rodeo events with the volume pitched up to full throttle, and you won't hear "What the heck are you doing! It's the middle of the night!"

You can sleep in the middle of the bed. In fact, *until* you can sleep comfortably in the middle of the bed you're still behaving like half a pair of scissors. Give me one good reason why you continue to curl into a still, quiet ball on the left side of the mattress. It's okay to spread out. Just shimmy over and enjoy the whole space. Grieving has its own time clock, which is different for each person, and you should take all the time you want, but it's perfectly okay to do it in comfort. More than that, it's your right. There are all sorts of things you can do to help yourself feel better.

You can wear your favorite ratty purple-plaid dressing gown now, the one with the hole in the elbow that your partner hated. And you never again have to eat that grim dinner of boiled corned beef and cabbage that your Irish in-laws insisted on dishing up every St. Paddy's Day. You can invite anyone you like for lunch or dinner whenever you want without having to clear it first with anybody except the invitee.

I *know* that you'd love to have your old life with your old love back—there's nothing you'd like more—but, hard as it is, it's healthier to try to focus on some of the positive things about being alone. If you allow yourself to become isolated and sink into serious depression, it's going to be a long climb back. Depression only has the power you allow it.

Another thing—telephones work two ways. You can't just wait for your phone to ring. Don't decide, because you're the newly alone person, that friends should be the ones to make that call. They did. And they have for weeks. However, after a while the ones that called you realized that you don't call *them* at times to say hello and see how *they're* doing. Maybe it's your turn to take the initiative to pick up the phone and reconnect with a friend.

You must know other widows or widowers and once-again singles that are probably feeling as transient as you're feeling. Perhaps they would be happy to have your dinner invitation. Not up to that? Then maybe you can manage an invitation for coffee or tea or a restaurant dinner. It gets easier once you decide to help yourself and make that first move.

But first of all, get yourself out of bed in the morning and out of your nightshirt. If you're a woman, you want to find your prettiest dress. Panty hose, a little blusher and eyeliner can't hurt either. And great shoes—lose the house slippers! A man knows what shirt and pants look best on him after he's groomed and ready to face the world. A smooth face and light aftershave; name me one woman who finds slightly musty, unshaved men in their undershirt appealing. Your friends want to see you at least try; they've missed you. Most of them understand what you're going through. They've been where you are now, and they know firsthand the grit and courage it took for them to get going again. They'll applaud your effort.

When you really feel up to it, there's probably a bunch of things you can do to make your life more comfortable. You can begin by handling a problem that's bugged you for years, something your partner refused to face. Maybe you'd love to tell your asbestos-tongued sister-in-law you no longer look forward to her criticism. She may not like you for telling her, but certainly she's going to watch her sharp tongue around you from now on. Claiming your own life can be a heady experience.

As much as you miss your wonderful sweetheart and mourn your loss, when you begin to look more positively at your newly single life, you'll know that you are going to be okay. You can count on it.

16

You Asked Him Out How Many Times?

Here's the situation: there's a great-looking widower new on the scene from Montana. His wife of twenty-five years died a couple of years back, and he's just bought a house in your neighborhood. Count on it, he'll be watched closely with acute interest by nearly all the unattached ladies in town. And why not. He's some kind of book-writing retired professor with the lanky build of an urban cowboy; he's also very funny and has both a clever mind and a healthy bank account. Plus he can't stand playing golf, and he doesn't go jogging at 4:30 AM. On top of all that, he loves to dance! For sure this man is first-class material.

Everything's perfect about the guy. But even if it weren't, the odds are in his favor to be popular, whatever his pedigree, in a gender-imbalanced population of older singles.

You think you'll ask him to a dinner party that you hadn't even planned to have until you met him at last night's fundraiser for the symphony. Actually, you might want to keep to yourself the part about arranging a dinner for the sole reason to ask him to your home. He also doesn't need to know how much you want to have your party first, before Olga (your best friend, also single, who is altogether too good-looking to have around him yet) gets back from Spain, suntanned and even better looking than when she left. Besides Olga is a terrible flirt and tries her wiles on every man, whether she likes him or not, just to prove, at age sixty-eight, she can still rope them in—a tendency that has lost her more than one woman friend.

It's now seven calendar months later and here's what has taken place:

1. He came to your first dinner party, and anyone could see he had a swell time mixing with everybody. He praised your cooking and loved what you'd done with your house.
2. Next you invited him to a weekend brunch. Again he was a great success—a real sweet guy and an entertaining conversationalist—an asset to any group.
3. The following week you arranged another dinner, and of course he was included. Truth of the matter is he wasn't just included, he was the reason you kept on having all the dinners and lunches and brunches for the weeks and months that followed. Friends were beginning to ask if the pair of you were a couple. But no. No, you weren't. In fact he never once phoned you between parties.
4. The only contact you had was when you called to invite him to your house or to accompany you to a gallery opening or the theater, or when you ran into him at the grocery store.
5. *He's basically shy*, you told yourself.
6. *He's still getting over his wife's death*—yet another excuse you gave him. Fact is you kept looking for excuses why he wasn't inviting you out.
7. *Why, oh why hasn't he made a move? Perhaps he was just too shattered when his wife died, and he's not ready yet to be involved again, and he needs more time?*

I doubt there's a woman alive who hasn't guessed and second-guessed why a man she is dying to date hasn't asked her out. Especially when she's made it obvious she's plenty interested to see more of him. What in hell is stopping him?

One afternoon I caught the *Oprah* show when she introduced former *Sex and the City* television scriptwriter Greg Behrendt to her audience. He'd just come out with a book to help women understand that if a guy you are nuts about doesn't ask you out it's because *he's just not that into you*. Behrendt was like a magnet to Oprah's mostly female audience; two hundred women visibly leaned forward to listen closely. He certainly had my attention as he talked about what to do if you really like a man who isn't asking you out.

Over the years he'd listened to a lot of girl-talk working on the hit TV series. One subject kept coming up in story conferences as possible material for the show: a woman agonizing through the same mating dance again and again about why a man she wants so badly to go out with hasn't asked her out. It was a recurring dilemma for the writers to sort out on the series. And it did not take place only on the show. Behrendt realized it was a situation that kept showing up in his real life outside the studio among his women friends.

Enough of this, he decided. It was plainly something women just didn't get, and he felt all those fabulous women putting so much energy and effort into men who weren't reciprocating begged an explanation. In his own circle of friends, the women he knew were savvy and beautiful, and he hated to see them wasting their time on guys who didn't respond to their keen interest and availability. Therefore, along with coauthor Liz Tuccillo, Behrendt wrote a book titled *He's Just Not That Into You.*

In his book he describes the no-excuses truth to understanding guys to women who just don't get it; there are no mixed messages.

Simply put, when a man meets a woman, no matter under what circumstances or however brief the encounter, he knows straight off if he's interested. He finds it rewarding to go after a woman who fascinates him, and he loves the chase. He was born to chase.

Men are hunters, they like to do their own hunting, and if it's you he wants, he'll find you. He doesn't need you to orchestrate his life. Greg says that you don't have to guess any longer why he didn't call you after you invited him to a dinner party or, a couple of weeks later, asked him to go to a movie. If you don't think you gave him enough time to know you, just look at how much time it took you to notice him and divide it by half. If he'd been interested when you met, he'd have booked you on the spot for a date. Behrendt's book is wonderfully warm and humorous. And enlightening. And very pro-women.

After Greg and Oprah had discussed his book and why he wrote it, a woman in the audience spoke up (I'm paraphrasing here): "So if he's not that into me, why does he seem happy to have me ask him to parties and special events? And why does he always say yes immediately to my invitations?"

"Because first of all he really does like you. Secondly he wants to keep you in his life in case he doesn't find anyone better."

"Wow, you don't pull any punches, do you?"

"No. And nor should you fool yourself. At gut level you know that he likes, maybe even admires, you, but he's not crazy about you. You don't need Zen insight for that. You may not like to admit it because you desperately want him to feel the same way about you that you feel about him right now. But it's no one's fault. The very best love between a man and a woman must have chemistry and it cannot be forced or fabricated or insisted on just because you want it. Another thing to know is that men are real wusses and don't want to tell a woman she's not the woman he really wants. He sure doesn't want to hurt her feelings, because he's a coward around weeping ladies, and he definitely doesn't want to answer a woman's questions about *why*. Or *what* she did wrong. No one did anything wrong!

"Listen to me. You are gorgeous. What I see when I look at you is a lovely woman, smart and sassy, a delightful lady any man with any sense would want to be around. That's not the same thing as a man seeing you as the only woman who captivates him, as the only woman in the world he knows he will ever want as his lady."

You will understand fully after reading *He's Just Not That Into You* that here is one writer who loves women and very obviously believes they deserve so much more than a rather charming fellow sopping up all their attention. His frank honesty makes such perfect sense that the fog will disappear from your vision with the realization that what you're doing by obsessing about a man who doesn't return your wholehearted affection is nothing more than an exercise in futility. And the only reason the man keeps accepting your invitations is because he likes you as a friend and you take him to great parties where he might meet another woman who completely bowls him over.

With Greg Behrendt's book to guide you, you'll quit wasting your time torturing yourself over any man who's clearly not smitten with you. Keep the thought that *your* Mr. Right is out there probably looking for you this very minute. Hold onto your emotional energy for when that right man comes along and makes it strikingly clear that he thinks you're the cat's pajamas and wants you to put him first in your thoughts from that moment on.

And what's wrong with that? Nothing. If you feel the same way about him, it can only be wonderful.

17

Facing Up to Alcoholism

Eileen punched the hot, damp bed pillow and threw one arm across her eyes to shield them from a mean sun that cut through her bedroom window, seemingly determined to add to her misery. A bitchy soccer team was kicking her brains savagely and using her eyes as goal posts; her hangover was only slightly smaller than Rhode Island.

But apart from feeling like she was going to die a violent death and join her ancestors in a matter of minutes, something else was pinching her conscience as she vaguely remembered a bar, a pay phone, and her own screaming crude language. "I must have phoned that rotten pig last night in Japan," she moaned into the pillow, "Oh, gawd, please say I'm only imagining things."

Her eyes flew open at the sound of the shower curtain being drawn. The bathroom door opened and a glare of hard white light spilled into the room, along with a splendid half-naked man who grinned sympathetically, flipped a wet towel onto the chair, and crawled into her bed. She'd never seen him before in her life.

Eileen yanked the sheet up to her chin. "What kind of fresh hell is this? Who *are* you?" No answer. "Do you know who you are?" she persisted. He looked at her in an odd way and shook his head.

"And I have no idea either, so that makes us even." Her stomach felt queasy, "I must be in a nightmare."

With as much control over her shakes and pounding head as she could muster, Eileen pointed to the pile of clothes on the floor, "Please get dressed." No reaction. "Por favor se pone la ropa?" Aha, jackpot!

She had no recollection of the man or where they met or how he ended up in her bed. Carl had walked out on her eight months earlier, and in that short time she'd sunk to slut status.

An hour later Eileen arrived at work. Huge black sunglasses over a jittery application of eyeliner and two slashes of blusher were the only extras with her skinny black sweater and black leather pants. She slid past the receptionist with a mumbled hello and ducked into her own cubicle to face a day of cold calling for property listings. All she really wanted to do was put her head down on the gray metal desk and sob. Her headache was brutal, her stomach rocky, and her legs unsteady.

Kate stood in Eileen's open doorway. "Bad night?"

"Carl's a bastard. I wouldn't be in this mess if he weren't such a lousy womanizer."

"One woman, Eileen. One woman who came along three years after you became a drunk."

Eileen's eyes watered up behind the dark glasses, "Do you always have to be so blunt? Can't you understand how hard it is for me to go from a married woman who didn't work, and hadn't worked for thirty-five years, to a divorced woman who has to have a job to make ends meet?"

"There are lots of us around. And, yes, I do understand perfectly well what it's like."

"Sorry. I forgot you're divorced."

"Lots of women are divorced. Did you also forget that my husband left for the same reasons that Carl couldn't take any longer? Or didn't you know that I used to be a drunk?"

Eileen was stunned. Personable, smart, sophisticated, whiz-of-an-office-manager-Kate—a drunk? "Why did you hire me if you thought so little of me?"

"Who said I thought so little of you? I knew you were in big trouble with booze when you walked into my office looking for a desk and a place to work. You aren't the first alcoholic I've hired. I'm going to put you on probation for three months: ninety AA meetings in ninety days. Take it, Eileen. You'll never have a better offer."

"I can't go to meetings every night for ninety days! Are you nuts?"

"If you don't like being sober after three months, you can leave this job and drink yourself to death if you want, but you'll do it on your own time, not mine." Kate turned around and went back to her front office.

Eileen sat at her desk shaking and scared; she felt completely out of her depth. She closed her eyes and tried to shut out last night's terrible scene in the back hallway of the bar; she saw her very drunk self, screeching long-distance threats into the pay phone. It was the second time she'd called Carl in such a state; the first call to Tokyo had cost her eighty-seven dollars and a migraine that lasted forty-eight hours. Her life was unworkable—she was facing a bleak future.

Eileen stared at the telephone on her desk. *AA? What the hell…* She let her breath out slowly and picked up the phone book. *It's really a no-brainer*, she decided. *I don't even have to know how to spell to look up the number.*

◆   ◆   ◆

Nine hours later she walked down the church basement stairs.

The hall was crowded with smilers and huggers and noisy with laughter; Eileen sneered inwardly at the whole happy mess and felt like killing Kate. *Where does she get off trying to control my life away from the office?*

At the far side of the room coffee and biscuits were set out on a long table. Eileen was dying for a coffee but wouldn't risk the chance of sloshing it all over the table in front of a bunch of reformed drunks. Her hands were shaking like crazy; she longed for the damned meeting to be over so she could get home and pour herself a decent drink. *This is going to be a lot harder than I thought. What if I can't do it? What if I end up being fired? I can't lose my job!* A tear slid out the corner of her eye and ran unchecked over a high cheekbone and into the cleft of her chin.

The speaker was in her mid-sixties, the same age as Eileen. She'd been a stay-at-home corporate executive's wife for forty years. Her story caught Eileen's interest, in spite of herself, because it so nearly paralleled her own experience. The woman wouldn't go to a restaurant that didn't have a liquor license. She didn't have a friend that didn't drink a lot; eventually she didn't have a friend left. She told the seated ex-drunks, "I paid no attention to my husband's threats, no attention to my grown children's arguments and tears over my drinking. I just cut them dead."

"My marriage, my family, my friendships, my interest in my husband's career, in the community, and in my home—everything that was once important became unimportant. There are few things that match the destruction an active alcoholic can inflict on a marriage. My self-worth dropped to zero at the same time I got to be snotty as hell."

How can she get up there and say all that stuff out loud? Eileen was amazed at her frankness.

"I think a Rent-A-Drunk service for a month would have been useful for my husband to test the appeal of a drunken wife before he married one." The speaker's last remark left her audience laughing out loud.

The laughter caught Eileen by surprise. *These people certainly have a strange sense of what's funny.*

As the group began to clear away the folding chairs in the hall, Eileen thought of all the times that she'd promise Carl to cut back on her drinking. Or to switch to white wine and pass on hard liquor—a tiring dance of her un-kept promises followed by arguments and threats that usually dissolved into tears and yet another round of promises. And more alcohol.

"First time at the group?" He was cute. Cute, fat, and bald, and putting the make on her—she knew the look.

Eileen nodded. "Yes, my first time." To herself she muttered, "And maybe my last time, too, creep."

A petite blonde in jeans and a white cotton tee grinned at Eileen and the bald guy, "Andy, leave her alone. She isn't aware of your killer ways with the ladies. I'm Bonnie," she took Eileen's elbow lightly, "and he's a letch. Dangerous man, he goes after all the best-looking new females." Bonnie steered Eileen away from Andy, who shrugged in good humor.

As Bonnie filled two cups with coffee, she introduced Eileen to a couple of women who were standing by the table. Eileen looked away and didn't acknowledge their hellos; quite suddenly she felt she wanted to go home. Bonnie quickly wrote a phone number on a paper napkin and gave it to Eileen. "Call me, please, just to say hello if you want, or to talk about how you're doing. I'll try to help." She didn't ask for Eileen's number, and she didn't ask her one single question or offer any unasked-for advice. Eileen liked her for that, and she tucked Bonnie's number into her shoulder bag and turned to leave.

Bonnie didn't try to stop her. She gave Eileen's arm a reassuring pat, "Call me if you need a lift tomorrow evening. No sense in taking two cars, and I'm going to be speaking, so I can use the support. You can keep me calm on the way to the meeting."

On the way home, Eileen tried to remember the last time anyone had offered her a phone number. She cringed as she thought of old friends who were fed up with her calls at two in the morning to bitch and weep about unfaithful, stinking, crummy husbands. Drunken phone calls in the middle of the night to people who didn't want to hear from her anymore.

She pulled into her driveway and dropped her tired head onto the steering wheel. This time there was no one to see the wash of tears streaking her cheeks.

♦   ♦   ♦

Bonnie was winding up her AA talk from a platform at the front of another church hall, her voice well modulated and clear, "In the car on the way home from an office party, my husband was giving me a hard time about my drinking. He was at his wits' end with me, but I was so smashed I was screaming at him to shut up giving me orders, and I grabbed the steering wheel and sent us straight into the cab of an oncoming truck.

"I didn't die as a result of my drunkenness, as a lot of alcoholics do in drinking-driving accidents, but Harry was killed." Bonnie's voice faltered, "Every day I live with the knowledge that I took away his life, but I still have mine, so I had better make my sorry existence count for something worthwhile."

Eileen sat very still in the front row trying to imagine what it must be like to wear that burden each day. In the car on the way to the meeting, Bonnie had congratulated Eileen on getting through the first twenty-four hours of sobriety. "It's fantastic! I'm so proud of you," she'd said, and it felt grand to get that boost of spirit, because her nerves were edgy after a very long sleepless night. Now Eileen wanted to find words to help Bonnie.

When the *thank yous* and *good nights* from the group were done and they were heading home, Eileen said, "I cannot imagine how difficult it must have been, Bonnie. You've come a long way; I admire that. What was the hardest part for you when you quit drinking?"

"Oh, no question about it—it was the physical stuff, first."

"Like not sleeping?"

"More like my nerves yelling at me to stop the funny business and feed myself a few shots of vodka to get things back to normal."

"I know what you mean. Right now I'm kind of guessing at normal myself. A couple of times last night I came so close to pouring myself a drink. I didn't think I'd get through the night. I couldn't sleep, my back was killing me, and I wanted to kick Carl any place it would do the most damage."

"What's the story there? Is he your husband? Are you still together?"

"Together? That's a joke. He had an affair with someone in his company—he's manager of Japanese/American sales for Texaco. I found out about it in a really ordinary way, a letter from his lover in a pocket of a suit jacket going to the cleaners, and it sent me on a five-day disappearing act to our cabin in the Adirondacks. Me and a case of Chivas—which I hate, but Carl always stocked it in the bar for business entertaining, and it was what I grabbed when I got the idea to run."

"He didn't know where you were?"

"I didn't tell him, that's true, but he had an idea where I might have gone. He phoned the caretaker, who came over and kept pounding on the door till I staggered over to open up and ask him to please leave me alone. I was crying and dirty, and I'd thrown up a few times. I was plenty scared.

"Carl drove up to get me. He'd called in a baby-sitter we'd used when our daughter came for visits with our grandchildren. His bags were packed and standing in the front hall when we got back to town. He handed me over to the sitter and left to catch a plane to Tokyo inside the hour. I can't believe what a rat he turned out to be. Thirty-five years together, and he treated me as if I was nothing. Absolutely nothing to him."

She wanted Bonnie to agree, but Bonnie said nothing; Eileen's shoulders began to tense up, and she was pretty sure Bonnie blamed her for being such a failure.

"Eileen, why did you come to AA? Was it your own idea to get help to stop drinking, or did someone give you an ultimatum—a courtroom judge, your boss, your kids? The reason I ask is because you seem, to me, anyway, to be good and angry, as if it's someone else's fault that your life is screwed up right now."

"Carl was my husband and a womanizer. I didn't screw up my life—he's the one that did the walking—he's the one who as soon as there was any kind of problem found another woman for himself, grabbed a plane out of the country, and left me to fend on my own."

"Are you saying that Carl made a practice of running around with other women? That he always walked away from a problem? That he never tried to help you to stop drinking?"

"That's too many questions," she glared at Bonnie. "And yes, he spoke to me about my drinking. He offered to pay for a rehab stay at Betty Ford a few years ago. He also said he'd take me to AA."

"Did he?"

"Did he what? Take me? No."

"Was it because he forgot or because he changed his mind? Or because you wouldn't agree to go?"

"Well, I certainly wasn't going to any rehab place, and I refused to have him march me into an AA meeting! I didn't need him to take me—he's not my father. I was sixty-two years old. He treated me like a baby!"

"Perhaps that's how he saw you. Look, I know how hard it is—not only to stop drinking, but to accept responsibility for the ways things happened. However, if you seriously want to stay sober, you're going to have to face a few truths. One of them is that Carl did not get you into a mess. But for now it's enough to admit that you're an alcoholic, and to not take that first drink."

Eileen saw that Bonnie was cutting through all her excuses. In her entire life she'd never come up against tough love, and she didn't think too much of it, either, when it was aimed at her. "I don't know that I can do it. I'm not good at doing difficult things."

"You'll have lots of loving support to draw on, but ultimately you are the only person to not pick up that first drink."

"What if I can't?" She felt miserable. It was easier to blame Carl than to face the fact that alcohol had her by the throat.

"But you *can* do it. I believe in you."

"At this point in time you're probably the only person in the world that is that much of an idiot," Eileen gave a shaky attempt at a laugh. "I may let you down."

"Not me—only I can do that. And you're the only one who can let yourself down. So you get some sleep if you can. It may be a week or so before you do, but don't fuss about it. Your body just has to get used to the new routine."

"Some routine, huh? I'll think of it as a new exercise tape."

◆   ◆   ◆

"My drinking only became a serious issue after Carl walked out."

"You mean it only became serious for you. But it must have been serious for others before then."

"What makes you say that?" Eileen asked sharply.

"Didn't you tell me that Carl had tried to get you to go to Betty Ford? The two of you were still together at the time, so you must have been drinking out of control before he left you, or he wouldn't have done it."

"Migawd, I hate it when you remember everything!" Eileen made a face at Bonnie.

"Well, Betty Ford is the top dry-out place in the United States, and it would have set him back a few thousand. I tend to remember big numbers and rich men."

"You're right. My drinking was out of control for a few years before he left me."

"One of these days you're going to have to thank him."

"Because *why?*"

"Because you wouldn't have hit bottom if he hadn't left. He protected you, but like you said yourself, you didn't want to be saved by him. That translates to 'you weren't ready.' He did the only thing to do when an alcoholic in his life wouldn't seek help—he walked away. Betty Ford, or anywhere else for that matter, couldn't have worked when it wasn't your own idea to look for help. Besides, an institutional setting is just another form of dependency—doctors and nurses to shoulder your problems."

"You're tough."

"You bet. And talking about tough, how hard has this past year been for you? Really, tell me."

"It certainly had its difficult moments, yet it's probably been the most exciting year of my life. You remember after I was just six months sober I told Carl I'd like to try to put our marriage back together?"

"Oh, do I! And when he told you it wouldn't happen, that's when I realized you were a lot stronger than I thought. It was amazing, actually, that I didn't have to pick you up off the floor after that slap."

"It's so weird to live with a man for thirty-five years and then find out it took him less than twenty-four weeks to replace me. By the time I spoke to him about a reconciliation, the two of them had already hired a preacher, and I belonged to yesterday."

"I know you're okay with it now, but back then it was rough. You've grown so much in the year. Besides, look at your life: you look fabulous, you're doing well in your job, your kids are talking to you, and you've made some wonderful new friends."

Eileen rummaged in her shoulder bag and retrieved her one-year chip that Bonnie had presented to her on her AA anniversary. "Others may see this as a plastic poker chip," she held it at arm's length to admire it, "but to me it's Olympic gold! A lot of the credit goes to you, I know that for a fact; I depended on you so much, and you were always there."

Bonnie flashed her a grin, "So what's the news you were bursting to tell me?"

"Well, true to Carl's high imagination, he came up with an idea that seems bizarre on the surface, but it really made sense the more I thought about it. In fact, in many ways he's working out to be more interesting as an ex-husband than he was as a husband. Are you ready?"

"Just say it!"

"I was trying to be dramatic, you ninny. Okay—here goes. Carl said that in his corporate life he gets to meet more well-heeled, decent, single, and single-again men than I do and that, if I agreed, he'd look at each possible man seriously and see that we met. His very words were, 'You deserve a good man, and I can help make that happen.' In other words, he offered to find me a husband."

Bonnie's eyes and mouth flew open and a strong laugh bubbled up in her throat. "Or he offered to become your pimp! I never heard anything like it! Ex-husbands don't behave like that."

"You know, at first I was insulted—or maybe it was hurt pride—but the more I thought about all of Carl's so-called wild ideas that worked well for him in business, the more I saw merit in his plan."

"But you're not a business. You don't think it's a little callous? He was your husband, for gawdsakes!"

"Actually I think it's quite sophisticated. I would like to meet suitable men. At this point in time, Carl respects me more than he has in years. Hell, I respect myself more than I have in a long time. And the reality is that in his position Carl does meet intelligent, interesting men who hold high-level positions in business; some are divorced, some widowed. He wouldn't put me together with a married man wanting an out-of-town date, I can trust him there."

"Then, if you and a man he introduces you to get hitched, he gets out of paying any kind of alimony, is that it?"

"That's part of it. A long time ago Carl taught me something I've never forgotten, and that is that any successful deal between two parties has to be mutually beneficial. In this case he may sound unfeeling or self-serving, but mostly it's practical."

"And odd. It's so damned odd it makes a certain kind of sense. After all he knows you better than anyone else. But you have to admit you were married to one arrogant man. Maybe he'll start a trend—a kind of pass-the-stick-in-a-relay-race-to-the-next-running-mate trend."

"I like the sound of a rite of passage better. Not too wonderful being referred to as a relay stick."

"When I think back to how you spoke about Carl in such a bitter way when we first met, and how mature and smart you are now, it's difficult to believe you're the same woman."

"Common sense deserted me totally when Carl walked out. I knew that I was in deep trouble with alcohol, and I was badly frightened when suddenly I was on my own without the prop of a husband. I damned him to hell and back to anyone that would listen. Pretty dumb."

"You're a lot of things, but dumb isn't one of them. Besides, the healthier you got, the less you cut him up. Muckraking doesn't suit you, but it does seem to be a specialty of too many divorced people, and not just women."

"We're a grim lot, I guess. Moreover if Carl was so terrible, then why did I stay with him all those thirty-five years? I was making myself look stupid. And if I were that stupid, what new man would be interested in having me in his life?"

"My guess is you were always smart—just that alcohol got in the way big time."

"Too true. Alcohol, the great leveler. As an alcoholic you really do give up control of your life to alcohol. And everyone around you gets hurt in the fly-past. It's a huge relief to regain my own life."

"So, what are you going to do about Carl's wild scheme? Going to go along with it?"

"Well, this is what I was dying to tell you: I already have! Joanna—that's Carl's new wife—had a few people over for brunch on Sunday, and Carl introduced me to the nicest man. His name is Bill; he's a widower of three years. Carl had spoken to him about me, and we got along from the minute he said hello. And I found it not only easy; I felt very comfortable. He's probably sixty-four, because he's going to retire next year, not too tall, steel gray hair, a really nice manner, and we laughed a lot; he looks directly at you when he's talking."

"Do you think he liked you?"

"Carl said he did; he called early Monday morning and gave me a report, then Joanna got on the line. She said Carl's plan is to give Bill two months to make something happen or we then move on to the next man. By "we" she meant Carl and herself! Isn't it weird? Anyway Joanna said, and I quote, 'I think it's a brilliant idea, but after all, Carl is so entirely brilliant.'"

Bonnie stared at Eileen open-mouthed, and Eileen stared back at Bonnie, then instantly and together, they cracked up, dissolving into one huge fit of unstoppable laughter.

18

For Men Only: get-with-it dating 101

Read the following to decide if you're old-fashioned when you take a woman out to dinner. You could be dating yourself if you do the following:

1. You read the menu out loud.
2. You call the waitress "my dear."
3. You ask your dinner date what she wants to order, and then you speak for her to the server: "The young lady will have the beef Stroganoff."
4. You mention that this restaurant was the one where you proposed to your first wife.
5. During the meal you exaggerate your dead wife's virtues and accomplishments or you complain at length about the witch of a wife who walked out on you.
6. You make remarks to your date laced with sexual overtones.

If you agree to even one of the above crimes, you are old-fashioned. Your date can probably read. The waitress is not your dear or your anything else, and she probably, quite rightly, pegs you as an old geezer.

Unless your dinner date has a severe speech impediment, she will, no doubt, prefer to ask the wait person about different choices on the menu and then order her own meal. And unless you're dining with your five-year-old granddaughter, your date is most likely not *a young lady* and doesn't see being called one a compliment. Besides, *young lady* is a patronizing term no matter what age. Don't allow yourself to become antique.

A saintly dead wife or the divorced wife of doom is not the wittiest topic of conversation. It's the lady you're with, not the one you're without, who should get your full attention. As for sexual innuendos: *way too much* physical pressure.

If guilty, drop these ridiculous habits and you can be a swell date.

19

Didn't Plan on Being Poor at Seventy

Who do you rely on most over the years? Who do you turn to when you're bursting to share something wonderful? Who advises you carefully when your life gets into an utter mess and you start behaving like a massive idiot and want to quit your responsibilities and run off to Morocco and say "to hell with everybody"? Your best friend, that's who.

Husbands, wives, and lovers come and go in a lifetime. It's not unusual, given the length of time that men and women last nowadays, that two or three long-term partnerships are fairly commonplace before you exit this planet for wherever better or worse place you're headed. But friendship—that's something else. A close friend can long outlast several marital or common-law relationships and remain a valued source of pleasure your entire life.

The following is an account of how two close friends each solved their own as well as each other's worrisome financial problems.

I know a fantastic woman in Montreal, Quebec, whose husband had a debilitating stroke that left him unable to dress himself properly or remember anything that had happened ten minutes earlier. He was left in this condition for seventeen years before his death. He'd owned his own business tuning concert pianos and grandly built church pipe organs; his career and his earning power were also finished the minute he suffered his brain accident. The strain of coping with a husband requiring almost total care affected Marie severely. She had to quit her part-time job, the earnings of which would not have adequately covered the costs of paid at-home care for Hector, to become his primary care giver herself.

As you can imagine, his long illness took a terrible toll on their emotional balance as well as on their savings. And after he died she took stock of her situation and decided it would be a struggle to continue to afford the gracious four-bedroom home they'd bought forty-five years earlier, when houses sold for much less money, and maintain the grounds and pay the property taxes that were steadily on the rise. The latest blow was a leaky roof that couldn't be ignored.

In her search for a solution to her finances she turned to her best friend, Tessa, who, now seventy-one, had been widowed a year longer than Marie. She, too, was struggling to meet expenses on her smart downtown address as she depended on little more than social security and a couple of small pensions.

The two concerned widows looked realistically at their separate situations and decided they could do better by combining their assets. Taxes, services, and maintenance on the two houses were eating a major chunk of their incomes. They hit on a great idea to have a substantially more comfortable future.

They decided to sell Tessa's house and live together in Marie's larger home. Tessa's small but trendy downtown location was appraised at the very same amount of money as Marie's large house that was in an older residential district. Tessa's house sold quickly to an eager young professional couple. With the proceeds she bought half of Marie's house. Instead of each woman owning a three-hundred-thousand-dollar house she could barely afford, they had papers drawn so that each legally owned half of Marie's house, freeing up one hundred and fifty thousand dollars for each woman. The extra money, sensibly turned over to a well recommended, certified financial planner, gave each of them some monthly investment income and eased their money headaches.

Marie chose a financial planner cautiously because she needed objective advice to make smart financial decisions. Anybody can call him or herself a financial planner: a banker, an insurance agent, or an accountant can claim that title. What she looked for was a fee-only, *certified* (meaning three years minimum experience) financial planner, a member in good standing with The Association of Financial Planners. (The AFP oversees financial planners much the same as the American or Canadian Medical Association is there to oversee certified doctors). This also gave her a controlling body to which she could address complaint should the need arise.

Within eighteen months Marie had a new man showering her with attention, but she also knew positively that, after her experience with Hector, she wasn't interested in marrying again. She felt she'd rather have a monogamous relationship than a second husband or, as some people say, a LAT (Living Apart Together) relationship, with separate houses and separate bank accounts. What she really wanted was to enjoy her new single life free of financial concerns without a possible burden of another ailing spouse.

There are other combined living arrangements that can work. Your quality of life can vastly improve if a group of older women and men friends, left in similar tight financial circumstances, pool their assets to buy or rent a large house together. By contributing their various skills, abilities, and talents (decorating, carpentry, painting, tiling, sewing, gardening, bookkeeping, cooking), they can all enrich each other's lives by sharing the costs and scheduled duties of a co-op house.

The thing that would likely be a prime concern would be having your own bedroom with an adjoining bathroom. There could also be personality problems if someone turned out to be a complainer or so dependent that she or he irritated practically the whole household. Is a seventy-eight year old flirt, who can't possibly open a can of sardines if there's a man around, a problem? No, that's just a bit silly, but anyone who always expects others to do his or her errands, or borrows money often and "forgets" to repay the loans—that's not good. By banding together in a shared home, you become a family unit in a way, and difficulties have to be addressed. Not to worry: most tricky situations can be solved sensibly in active group discussion.

I don't think you need a special license to create a casual co-op situation, just a well thought out written agreement between participating housemates. But perhaps in areas of uncertainty (important areas such as how to proceed in the case of serious physical or mental illness or death), it's best to have a binding contract. You can ask a lawyer to have a look at your agreement or perhaps draft one for you. AARP (American Association of Retired Persons), and CARP (Canadian Association of Retired Persons), have lists of lawyers who volunteer their time and advice to members in need of consultation in various parts of the country.

If your are in a tight position financially, you might think of speaking with one or more good friends on fixed incomes whom you know are also concerned about cash flow, about the idea of shared housing. Friends can help friends in important ways and end up helping themselves at the same time.

If you don't actually know someone who is interested in joining forces, a well-written ad for a housemate, along with a face-to-face interview and a thorough check of references, could prove workable.

The National Shared Housing Resource Center was developed as a resource for persons interested in exploring alternative housing arrangements whereby two or more unrelated people share a dwelling, each retaining a private space within the dwelling. For a growing number of persons struggling to keep housing costs within their budget, shared housing is an affordable and viable option. The NSHRC Directory provides names of regional coordinators, with national and international contact numbers (phone, fax, e-mail and snail mail addresses). On the Internet, you can Google: National Shared Housing for information pertaining to your locale.

20

Screw Impotence!

Are you alone again and fearful of becoming deeply involved with a new woman with whom you might not be able to have coital, or what you may think of as normal, sexual relations? Are you nervous about the fatal day when she discovers the embarrassing truth of your sexual impotence that you find utterly shameful?

Please hear this: it does not mean that you cannot love a woman or that she cannot love you back, nor does it mean you cannot make love to a woman.

I know a well-kept secret. It's kind of unspoken classified information among too many older women—they're simply thrilled with the prospect of an impotent man in their later years because they're fed up with whole sex issue anyway! Perhaps they never liked it very much.

Imagine that. Here you are with man's biggest torment since Adam lost his rib, limp with worry over an uncooperative body part that bothers you more than your family's welfare, your jowls, your thickening waist, or your stock market portfolio. Yet, all the time you were suffering needlessly, because for one reason or another, huge numbers of older women don't give a hoot about it.

But don't give up! Other healthier women, less self-involved, know how to handle impotence and are natural and willing sex partners with their lovers; to them impotency will never be a critical issue that blocks intimacy.

Of the two kinds of women who don't find impotency a problem, one kind has always run on a low flame; if her partner is chronically impotent, there's a sigh of relief from her side of the bed. This kind of woman wouldn't be in the least upset with your inability to have coital sex or any other kind of sex. "Thank god!" she'd say (though probably not out loud). Vaginal dryness is blamed for her reason to give up on sex altogether, even though there are countless ways of eliminating vaginal dryness in order to give and receive sexual gratification. More likely she wants sex in any form to be in her past—in your past, too! She'd prefer to concentrate on her bridge game or a stray cat. If a relationship without sex is what she's after, you can expect that the nearest you'll get to intimacy is her interest in your blood pressure, cataracts, and chiropody. But somehow lengthy conversation about bunions and the best buy in strong toenail clippers isn't romantically satisfying.

The other kind of woman, a lustier lady, is what you really wish for this time around—an enthusiastic partner who's always enjoyed sex and finds romping it up with her man exhilarating. She will never accept a life without it. With her you can find a very private, sensuous, at times vulnerable life you only thought was the stuff of fantasy. There's hope for that poor demented member after all.

If you're in your late sixties or seventies, give or take a few years, chances are you'll be interested in dating a woman around your own age. I can assure you that any woman in that age bracket knows the score on impotency. She's most probably had a former husband or lover who was impotent occasionally, if not chronically. It's not going to throw her into hysterics. The University of California–Berkley has published statistics stating that more than ten million American men are chronically impotent. The information and numbers cited were taken from reported cases of patients seeking help from their doctors, but the true numbers that would include unreported cases are most certainly higher. Advertisements for Viagra state there are over forty million men occasionally or chronically troubled by sexual dysfunction in the United States alone.

The University of California's Wellness Letter, a monthly publication, listed the following percentages: by age fifty-five, 18 percent of men report the problem; by age sixty-five, the figure increases to 30 percent, and by the age of seventy-five, some 55 percent of the male population report suffering from impotence. In this last group of seventy-five year olds, I strongly suspect the percentages of impotent men are higher, and some guys are likely exaggerating their performance. Yet not all of them want to jump over a cliff.

A lucky man has a vital woman in his life, a lady who simply adores him and fully understands that when he's happy in bed, all's right with his world. That includes her world, too. Now that you find yourself once more single, you're in a position to choose a new partner with whom you have a decided positive-chemistry connection. You must look for that woman.

Impotency isn't for sissies, and an impotent man can only make himself totally miserable if he pre-decides that he can't start over again with another woman and make her happy. A man and a woman of any age who are crazy about each other will find ways to express themselves intimately. Sex is a robust life-giving force, as unstoppable and instinctive as breathing. Working with impotency is nothing more than a challenge. It's where a loving couple gets inventive. Believe it, dizzy lavish sex at any age is available with the right partner.

21

Time to Toss Drunks, Married Lovers, Liars, and Moody Jerks

So long, drunkie!

There are few things that match the destruction an active alcoholic can wreak on a marriage.

Don't get the idea that you can save a drunk, either. Only a drunk can save her or himself. Cutting down consumption doesn't work. Changing brands doesn't work. Beer or wine instead of hard liquor—forget it! It's just a joke, and not even a funny one.

It doesn't matter how clever, how creative, how funny, how charming a person is, nothing works to stop an alcoholic except total abstinence. And if the person in trouble won't consider abstinence, then all the cleverness, creativity, humor, and charm cannot prevent slaughtered relationships, damaged health, and, if the addiction isn't dealt with, death. The only thing to do if an alcoholic in your life won't seek help is to walk away.

A word of caution here: never threaten an alcoholic with an ultimatum if you aren't prepared to carry it out (i.e., never threaten to leave if the drinking doesn't stop entirely unless you are fully prepared to do so).

Not wanted: married lovers who pass as bachelors

A married lover in your single-again life is your own business if you're into time-shares and can handle the situation, and you're not hoping for this person to become a permanent partner. But a married lover who *lies* about being single is not good for the soul.

Let's say you're a woman with a niggling suspicion that the man you're falling in love with is married, complete with a flock of kids and grandchildren whom he hasn't mentioned. For the sake of all involved, you may want to determine the true picture.

Before you go shooting off the Richter scale, ask him to be truthful with you. If he insists he is single, but you still don't believe that he's telling the truth, you can make some phone calls to people who know him. If you find out he is married, you then have your answer, and that's the end of the guesswork, and no doubt, the end of the relationship.

But suppose you've got it wrong, and he's perfectly legit. Once he becomes aware of your poking, you'll probably have damaged the relationship irretrievably. Consider carefully your need to know. If you feel you want a future with this man beside you, you *do* need to know his status.

Or take this situation: a man you're falling for is from another city or another country; you've not met his family, and he never refers to them. His background isn't known to you or to your friends, and he doesn't seem to have friends of his own. It all seems kind of peculiar and makes you uneasy. He never uses a credit card. Is this because his credit is bad? Or is it that he can't risk a traceable record of purchases? He's rarely available evenings, only occasionally on Saturdays, and never on Sundays. He comes to your place; you haven't been invited to his place. You imagine things. You probably do have reason to be seriously apprehensive. There are some very simple things you can do.

Start with the telephone directory, and call his listing when you know he's not at home. (How could he be at home when he's belting Cole Porter lyrics in your shower at this very minute?) If the phone is picked up at the other end by a woman, ask quickly if you're speaking to Mrs. Blah-blah, the wife of your wet lover. Actually, you might just leave that last bit out for now; but don't jump the gun simply because a woman answers. It could be his mother. Yes, it could. So ask the lady, "Are you his mother, his daughter, or his wife?" It's that simple.

Perhaps he has an unlisted phone number, or you don't know exactly where he lives. A city directory, at the reference desk of a public library, will give you his street address if the house is registered in his name. You can drive by and ask one of his neighbors down the street if they know where Mrs. Whatever-his-surname-is lives. "Is it his wife or mother who lives there?" "Both," the neighbor says. "Oh, my," you say.

If he's mentioned a golf or racquet club, you can easily find out if he and a wife are members. Call the club and ask if Mr. and Mrs. Judas Iscariot (substitute his real name) are members. You might sense some hesitancy from the club steward to give out membership information; just say that you're supposed to meet them for dinner at their club tonight, but you're not sure if you have the right club.

Is he retired? If not, then I assume you know where he works? If you call and reach his secretary, tell her that it's his wife (with a bad cold—cough heavily) and ask to be put through to your husband's office. This could be a shock for him if another thing you weren't told is that he has a dicky heart!

It's smart, and it's right, to check out nagging suspicions, but *only* if you're heading into a serious romance with that person, because if you allow yourself to get involved with a dishonest married man and later claim to be his victim, it doesn't wash. If you allow the idiocy of a weak relationship, then you are both wrong: him for lying, and you for ignoring your instincts. The outcome of your relationship is entirely your own responsibility.

It can happen the other way around, too, where a man is the one deeply involved in a situation where he suspects a woman who he's been seeing steadily isn't being straight with him. He feels she might be married.

A sea of information is available to anyone upon specific request: voter's registration lists, property records, and licensing records for a car, a boat, a business, or a house. You can also examine the following: death certificates, records of marriage if those particular records are considered to be in the public domain in a particular state or province. Divorce documents are filed in the county where the divorce took place. It's amazing and halfway disgusting that most of this recorded data is so handily available to the public simply by using a computer on a front desk counter at city hall, without even divulging your own name. Even criminal activity data, if you have the patience to search for it year by year, is entered on a city hall computer that anyone can access. If you live in a small town, you may have to go to the nearest city in the same state or province to access the information.

It's not enough that you're wildly curious. Absolutely none of your investigation is valid unless you're sincerely considering marrying or going into a business partnership with the woman about whom you harbor upsetting misgivings: her "stories" sound farfetched and her reasons why you're not invited to her apartment sound fishy. Her only phone is a cell phone. She doesn't talk about either her family or the past. She's evasive about her whereabouts when you're not together.

When in doubt, check it out. If you truly want to be a team, it's acceptable for you to get to the truth if she won't face your questions. For everybody's sake go easy; there may be very good reasons why she's withholding parts of her life. Perhaps she's the victim of a stalker or a vicious ex-husband. Or is it too much of a stretch to imagine that she could be in the Witness Protection Program?

For me it is.

An added thought: if you've *knowingly* got yourself involved with a married woman, or a married man, fallen in love with that person, and now want to know if your lover will ever leave her, or his, spouse—get real. Just the fact that you had to ask, you likely already *know* the answer.

Unexplained moodiness is unfair

A mistake is a mistake. But unless he twisted your arm painfully on purpose, and you'll be in physiotherapy for months to come, then you have to figure out if what he actually said or did was really as terrible as you're making it out to be. You've each been married before; you both should know how to resolve conflict. Moodiness is not an option.

When you fell into your all-consuming dark mood, were you already sore about another situation where your feelings were badly hurt? Do you have a list of complaints that you can't drop, that you feel he doesn't recognize or understand? Is keeping it to yourself helping the situation?

Whatever it was that wound you up, you want to identify it and deal with it, because unresolved problems rankle; they will reappear and eventually destroy your ability to enjoy life, together or separately.

You may have behaved in a moody manner during the entire course of your first marriage, and here you are starting out with a new man and you're up to the same old tricks. Injustice-collecting is for the very young; it's also unbelievably unproductive.

Instead of you thinking that he should know what he's done wrong, and that he should do something about it, try telling him what got you so upset. He cannot second-guess what's in your mind, because he has no idea what's in your mind. Men and women are different species. They no more think alike than do a giraffe and a tulip.

You have to tell him. Keep your voice reasonably calm and don't go crazy on him, because a man is totally at sea when a woman hits him with flying accusations of the never-ever-always ilk.

You like this man, remember that. Give him the opportunity to put things right, to straighten out the problem, the same problem he probably didn't even know existed until you went deadly silent and sullen.

Moodiness really is a crashing bore. Youngsters are allowed to get away with it occasionally because they don't as yet have the verbal skills to explain their feelings, but that's not the case here. Have you ever been around someone who quit talking to you but wouldn't explain why? Remember how it felt?

When there's a real or imagined concern that's serious enough to send you into nervous-making, tension-ridden silence, you've created a situation where you have those inside-your-head conversations with your partner where he will always lose and where you, too, will lose. Nothing gets resolved in those interior monologues where you control the entire exchange.

The longer you remain stubbornly tight-lipped, the harder it is to confront the original problem, which is now compounded by your punitive silence. Clearly the silent treatment is a poor choice, and so far all you've done is complicate it further. Try to sort it out fair-mindedly.

Fair-minded means just that; there are two people to consider here. Say what's bothering you; you need to be listened to in full. Tell him what upset you, then, let him explain his side of the situation without interruption from you. Once you've listened to his story, hopefully you can both apologize and have the grace to put it behind you. It's over. A problem that's over should remain over and not be brought up in a litany of complaints each time a new situation arises.

22

Never Let Yourself Be Degraded

You're kind of new at living on your own, and you feel lonely without a partner to share your life. When you're lonely, in fact *especially* when you're lonely, is when you have to be on guard about allowing anyone to treat you poorly. *Anyone* is **not** better than no one if that person is unkind or ignorant of your feelings.

This is a "run, don't walk" situation: get away fast from anyone who undercuts your confidence to make you feel uncomfortable. The need to degrade someone is a form of dominance that can begin as mild criticism by a person who wants you to do things his or her way instead of your own way. The demands most always get more severe over time. And you never win because the goal isn't to better you; it's to belittle you.

With a remark such as, "Why don't you do something about your weight; you look like a beached whale," your partner was totally disrespectful. And when you objected to that cutting remark, you were told, "Stop being defensive; it was constructive criticism." Don't you believe it! You do not have to put up with cruel rudeness from anyone.

Let's look again at that remark about your weight and how it was said: Was it said in front of others in a cynical way to get a laugh? And why did you have to be humiliated by a person you cared about, who later swore it was supposed to be all in fun, no apology given? And on top of this, you were further insulted with "Where's your sense of humor?" There's a term for this sort of behavior; it's called *leveling;* it's what a coward does to your self-esteem when he tries to reduce you to his level.

If the relationship is important to you and, in your mind, worth saving, you need to have a serious conversation about criticism, the need to control, and the issue of degradation. Do keep in mind, however, that this situation is unlikely to improve, because obviously an ignorant fool is an ignorant fool, and if you had to explain that it was an ugly degrading remark, there's probably no hope for change.

Trust your instincts. Believe in yourself. Spend more time with positive people and in time you'll find a good partner. You do not belong in a relationship with a hurtful person who tries to diminish you.

23

He Didn't See Her Coming

Historically, we've heard and read multiple stories about men conning women (especially older women), for money, for property, and for sex. Women have been loudly outspoken on the damage and humiliation they suffered. Men, however, are seemingly more embarrassed by anyone knowing they were duped by a conniving woman, and are loathe to admit they got taken.

But sure, men get conned by women. Lots of men have fallen prey to conniving women; usually the common denominator in the victim's personality is a lack of worldly wisdom or informed judgment. And loneliness. Loneliness is truly the main hook on which a guy who's likely to be conned can hang his heart.

During the 1940s Susanna Mildred Hill, a sixty-year-old mother of ten kids, was a famous American lonely hearts scam artist who bilked hundreds of men out of thousands of dollars in gifts and money by convincing them that she was a gorgeous, badly abused twenty-year-old girl. In her heart wrenching, beautifully written letters to lonely men advertising in the personal columns, she became a noble soul seeking a man to save her from a dreadful fate. She needed cash sent to a postal box so she could escape her tormentor.

Mildred Hill became immortalized in books, but there are plenty of other women in the business of conning men. One older man I heard from in my research told me he gave Andrea, a sweet-talking female member of a telephone dating service, money to complete her education. She claimed she hated most of the men who subscribed to the telephone service, as all they wanted to talk about was crude sex, but she had to do it because she had no marketable skills and couldn't get anything any other work after her husband left her destitute with a small child. Only a naive man could fall for that one; Andrea knew she had a real gullible guy on the line. They talked nightly on the phone, and he wanted desperately to help boost both her circumstances and her feelings of self-worth. Oh, she was good at it—the lady-in-distress scheme, the oldest scam in the book—and she had him begging to send her money.

Andrea wanted cash only sent to a private mailbox service. Never a check, she warned, in case her insanely jealous former husband would trace it and come after him and beat him up; according to Andrea, her ex was stalking her. She told her same tale to many many men and collected several thousand dollars before she was reported to the police by one of her victims who became suspicious.

Even though it's a striking blow to your pride to accept it, perhaps you, too, have been duped by a conniving woman who claimed to be someone she definitely wasn't. You're certainly not the first, nor are you likely the last man to be taken in by a pro. You surely recall this scene that took place shortly after your wife's death when you were simply too naïve and heartbreakingly lonely to recognize what was going on: you were introduced to Dorothy at a town hall taxpayer's meeting. She was a striking woman whom you never imagined in your wildest moments could be interested in you. This classy lady made an immediate impression with her air of quiet confidence and charm that put everyone around her at ease. She probably could have had her pick of any man, but for some amazing reason she chose you. It felt good. It wasn't her looks alone, not by a long shot; it was her sincerely affectionate manner and obvious joy at just being with you that mattered most; soon after you met you were inseparable.

She promised a warm future: she whispered sexy words, talked about New York City with just the two of you, a water bed, and a huge bottle of mayonnaise, things you never expected to hear at your age.

She said she'd never felt so attracted to, so perfectly right and in tune with, any other man in her whole life as she did with you.

What a great feeling, and how lucky you felt with her adoring attention. Her attitude of looking to you for advice and assurance made you feel eight feet tall. One evening as you waited in the ticket-purchasing line at the movie theater she told you the lease was up on the three-year-old Honda she drove, and she either needed to renew the lease or purchase the vehicle. You offered to foot the bill. "But I've had trouble with that car," she said, "and would rather own a new Lexus, something solid I can depend on. Could you really do that for me? You can? Really?" she shrieked when you nodded, grinning at her excitement as she wrapped her arms around you in the theater line-up and everyone around you cheered. "Omigawd, I've never known anyone so wonderful as this beautiful man," she told the onlookers. That was on Thursday night.

The sleek silver gray Lexus was purchased off the showroom floor the next morning, and later that evening she wowed you exuberantly with uninhibited sexy moves, sending you home with a broad grin on your face early so she could get a good night's beauty sleep.

Six o'clock Saturday morning she drove off in the newly-registered-in-her-own-name Lexus and hasn't been heard from since.

The super at the condo where she lived told you she'd taken her furnished unit under another name on a three-month lease. The lease was up the Saturday she took off. Her closets were bare, and the woman you knew as Dorothy, her suitcases, and the brand new Lexus were gone. Everything gone. Poof.

"What could I have done differently?" you asked, heartsick, ashamed, and feeling like a moron.

Learn much more about her. Not every woman who needs occasional financial help is a con, and you don't want to stop trusting women in general, but in this particular case, she robbed you big time, and she's the one who should be ashamed, not you.

24

Grown Children Angry Over Their Parents' Divorce

"I don't want to hear it."

"And why not? You seem to think you can bring your problems to me, but it doesn't work the other way around?"

"That's exactly right. You're my mother for gawdsake! I really do not want to know about your problems with your new boyfriend," Andy's voice over the phone was firm. He was so damned sure of himself.

"Do you give the same limits to your father and his little bimbo?"

"That's what I mean. Hell, you wanted out of your marriage. You split up the whole family, and yet you never miss the opportunity to put down Dad or his girlfriend, who, I might add, you've never even met, and who is not a bimbo."

"Oh, you like her, is that it? Well, you would, I guess—twenty years younger than good-old Dad; she's more your age than his age," Ceecie shot back in anger.

Andy started to say something but checked himself. At forty he probably felt he didn't want to get involved in a shouting match with his mother. "I'll call next week. Julie wants you to come for the twins' birthday," Ceecie could hear him hesitate, "alone. Please, Mom. It'll be just family. Dad is also invited."

Ceecie couldn't answer.

"Mom? Come on. Don't do this."

She heard the break in her own voice when she said, "Sure, Andy. You can count on me. Too bad the reverse isn't true." Slowly she laid down the receiver.

When the line went dead, Andy, too, probably hung up and muttered, "Damn it. I sure hope I never do this to my kids."

Ceecie stared at nothing in particular for a couple of minutes. Then she got out of bed, wandered into the living room, and sank into the amiable, faded linen roses of her old sofa. She let her head fall back onto a soft eiderdown-filled cushion.

She already felt lonely and oddly unsure of herself; she felt defeated emotionally, and she had less available money than at any time in her adult life. *The last thing I need is disapproval from my own children*, she thought. But she had to acknowledge the fact that both Andy and Joscelyn, her daughter, were plenty hurt over the divorce.

Ceecie sat there turning things over in her mind: *The kids hate the fact that Dan and I once loved each other but no longer do. They're sad and still angry that I left Dan. Take today for instance—the phone call from Andy had started out all right.* "Hey, Mom. Did I wake you? I called early because I thought you'd be working in the garden later."

"It's okay. I'm still in bed, but I've been awake since five thirty. Luke and I had plans for the day, but he changed his mind when an old friend of his called and wanted to play golf. I don't even know if it's a man or woman friend. He's done it before." And that's when Andy told her he didn't want to hear about her problems with her new boyfriend.

Earlier in the week she'd told her therapist, "It means nothing that my kids are grown up and on their own. Their lives are turned upside down by my decision to divorce, and I know that it's vital that I listen to what they have to say on the matter without interruption and, above all, without becoming defensive."

"But you don't have to agree with them. Nor should you allow either of your kids to become abusive of your feelings," the therapist answered. "At any age—teen to fifty—the self-centered side of a child's personality can, and often does, come forward over a parental divorce. Children of any age resent their lives being upset by a decision that spikes their comforts. Their lives are being disrupted without their permission and, no matter how tempted you are to explain yourself, they do not want to be embarrassed by listening to your side of the divorce equation nor forced to take sides."

Ceecie closed her eyes against the brilliant sun streaming in through the living room window; she felt a migraine coming on. *Well, I failed with flying colors today! I should bite my tongue before I stoop to cynical remarks or hang up abruptly—because as far as the kids are concerned, the blame for the split is mine, and they don't want to hear anything about my personal problems.*

When she and Dan first separated she had tried to talk with her daughter, but Joscelyn stopped her cold. "You caused this mess and you can handle it. If you need counseling, I'm not available; you'll have to buy it from a qualified psychologist." The word "daughter" took on a whole new meaning for Ceecie. Joscelyn, who poured out her soul to her mother regularly over any minor tragedy of her own, was not available. It hurt.

However, the therapist had agreed with Joscelyn's reasoning, if not her manner. "Steer clear of any talk of your ex's shortcomings. If you have nothing good to say about your former mate at this very stressful time in all your lives, keep quiet. And never use your children for counseling. Your daughter is dead right on this one: it is your mess, and you *can* handle whatever it is you have to handle. They have quite enough on their plates right now trying to sort out their own feelings."

"I didn't marry Dan, and we didn't have a family together, with the notion to give it a sporting couple of decades then spring for a divorce. But it happens. Life happens."

"If your marriage was unfulfilling and unfixable, your children must be told that. Whether or not they approve of you, you are not going to stay with their other parent just to please them, because while they're off living their own lives elsewhere, you'll be the one left in a loveless situation," the therapist glanced at the wall clock. "Your kids have one kind of relationship with their father. Your own relationship to that same person, however, was an intimate one and not a situation to be discussed with your children of any age. And that goes double for any thoughts you might have of asking for their attention about new boyfriend problems."

"All I need is for them to understand that it's my business who I love. It's also very much my business who loves me."

"You can tell them that. But it will take time for them to accept it. There's no rush. Behind all the anger and hurt there's a solid relationship between you and your grown children. Hold onto that thought and just try your best. In the process, you'll probably fall on your face a few times and feel terrible."

Remembering the therapist's words, she decided to stop punishing herself. A quick call to Andy to apologize helped both of them.

Ceecie replaced the receiver and stared into the cheeky eyes of a framed photograph of her ex-husband sitting on the desk. "You, on the other hand, are going into a box in the basement where you can grin at all the other snapshots of yourself in the same crate. How come I took so many pictures of you? Why didn't you take any of me?"

25

Concerning "Formers" and "Exes" (and why to keep your mouth shut about them)

Are you an intelligent, decent man responsible for support payments each month to a former wife of many years? If you find it's a struggle financially, and especially if you hope to have another wife someday and don't plan to be chronically poor, think about this: how about introducing your ex-wife to suitable available men? Tell all the guys how amazing she is. If you concentrate hard, you'll find a perfect match. Who better to know?

Speak about her with respect and good humor in public; rubbishing an ex-wife is tacky and no one wants to listen to it, so keep your private irritations private. Your sophistication will be noted, and your generous attitude is a healthy legacy to adult children of that former marriage. Besides, you could be looking at a big bonus of getting her off the alimony list if you find her a wonderful new husband. A wonderful, rich new husband is smarter still.

Along the same principle, if you're a savvy divorcee, you'll be smart to be loyal socially to your former husband. Privately you may wish the old womanizer permanent impotence, but public slime throwing has never had hygienic overtones. And your kids—even if they're adults themselves—don't need to hear how their dear dad was a rotten, two-timing walking phallus.

Moreover if he was so terrible, then why did you stay with him all those thirty years? Were you crazy, or what? And if you were that crazy, what new man would be interested in having you in his life now? It really is a lot wiser to keep old marital dirt to yourself.

Widows and widowers are alone again under different circumstances. But isn't it a riot how most widows and widowers insist they had just the most perfect marriages that ever were? Could this be true? Surely you'd have to be barking mad not to be skeptical in some instances.

But even if those old marriages were ideal, the constant reference to a dead saint of a husband or wife is a way of telling a new person in your life that he or she doesn't quite measure up. Who can match wits with iconic perfection, an object of uncritical devotion? And a dead one at that! Who wants to?

A widower implies that his wife was a paragon instead of the woman who he loved dearly in spite of a few flaws. He's forgotten the time he had to have stitches when she threw a brass pot at him.

A widow speaks of her irrecoverable husband as a model of excellence in spite of his questionable habit of patting every woman's rear end within reach, which was so hard to deal with when he was alive.

Comparing a new person in your life with a retouched image of a dead mate will guarantee isolation from warmth and intimacy. Is a reality check in order?

26

When Your Lover Exhibits a Violent Temper

And when she or he storms out the door in a blistering rage—this one's way too easy—you shut and lock the door. No one has to tolerate a filthy-tempered friend or lover.

This sad first-person account is from Francie, a British woman presently living in America, in Washington State: I'd been seeing Judd for several months. It was going so well—we were really loving it. At sixty-eight we each had a few conceits and irritating habits, but we had many more positive things in common: we both practically ate books, we enjoyed movies, live theater, jazz, opera, museums, restaurant dinners together as well as meals with friends. He was a better cook than I. We loved sailing together on Puget Sound and we both adored island travel—Bali, Hawaii. He, an unbending Republican, and me, a spirited Democrat, assured hot debate, yet we listened closely to one another's ideas. He didn't take argument of his opinion easily, but our conversation was always lively and we laughed a lot together; that was one of the best parts.

Separately we each had stimulating friends and a family of adult children and grandchildren with various successes and failures behind them. Between the two of us, we'd stacked up a few failures and successes of our own in old relationships and careers. In other words we'd each led a full life before we started dating, and neither of us would have welcomed a partner who was in any way a dud.

One day, after a particularly hilarious morning where he was trying to teach me to tango in the kitchen, he had to get going for a five o'clock business meeting in Seattle. Since he would be having a very late dinner, I offered to make him a sandwich to eat in his car. He turned down my offer.

"But I can make it while you're getting dressed," I suggested.

"No, I'll be fine, don't bother."

"It's no trouble, really. How about cheese and ham?"

And, as Francie reported, that's when all hell broke loose: Inside the length of one measly second, perhaps even less, he swung around abruptly, his body stiff with anger, and turned mean and ugly. It was so quick it was absolutely astonishing. I still can't quite believe it happened. Or even why it happened.

He started screaming at me, "I told you I do not want a sandwich! Can you not understand simple English?" In a flash his voice shot to a threatening level. "You have no idea who you're dealing with! So stop insisting on a damned sandwich that I don't want." His face, unnaturally red and flushed from what sounded to me like a lifetime of injustice collecting, was filled with contempt, and his rigid, shaking finger was inches from my face. "Don't ever, *ever* tell me what I want! No one tells me what I want!" His ugly, near-falsetto screeching ruled the moment. Along with his boiling rage, the tension he created was sickening; he was completely out of control. And worse, I could see there was no way he wanted to calm down; he was reveling in throwing his weight around. So I left the room—a tantrum's only a tantrum if someone's there to witness it.

Of course you know it really had nothing whatsoever to do with a ham sandwich, Francie continued in a voice flattened by sad recollection: Ten minutes later he came into the living room where I was seated with a book; I wasn't reading it, the damned book was simply a prop, at best a wobbly prop. He knelt beside my chair to thank me sweetly for one of the nicest days he'd ever had. Did I hear correctly? This man was badly disturbed and he was in my house; it was as if he'd flicked a personality button to become Mr. Nice Guy again, and truly that scared me more than his vile temper.

I asked him what happened back there in the kitchen to make him so vicious and told him I wouldn't tolerate that kind of behavior. Omigawd! Immediate frenzy. He went berserk all over again when I said I wouldn't tolerate his behavior; he was completely beside himself that I'd criticized his unhinged ranting. He leapt to his feet, grabbed his keys and jacket, roared out of my house, and took off wildly in his car.

Immediately I shut and locked the door behind his dramatic outburst and exit, because instinctively I knew what an unleashed temper could turn into; I sensed I'd narrowly escaped physical violence as I sank into the living room sofa, dumb with relief.

I'd never witnessed a ridiculously infantile tantrum in a grown man. I'd never seen the mercury rise from decent to reckless in seconds flat. In fact he was no longer a grown man when he was shrieking mad; in my mind he'd become a pompous cartoon. Any man who is about to enter his eighth decade of life and still behaves like an ass is pathetic.

His blazing ego, however, was clearly acceptable to him, because when he called a few days later to say he didn't like to leave things hanging between us, he was deadly quiet when I stopped him. "You can stop right there because there is no *us*, Judd. Anything good between us you destroyed absolutely with your savage temper."

There was no way I would ever trust him again with my emotions, yet at the same time I also felt he had to be quite concerned about his fragile posturing and plenty worried about his own erratic conduct. I told him about a truly reliable psychologist who'd helped me with problems following my divorce, a man who works exclusively with creative neurotics, possibly a good contact for him because almost certainly I wasn't the only person to have been on the receiving end of his flash mood swings. But he flatly refused outside help. "I am what I am," was his answer.

What he was was way too neurotic for me, not because he had problems, but because he made a rotten decision to do nothing about them.

I could see how badly Francie had been hurt by someone dear to her. But whether it's mental, physical, or emotional abuse, it doesn't matter; it's not safe, not secure, and it doesn't make him less of a bully that he didn't actually haul off and hit her. What made her story doubly sad was that it didn't have to happen. There are therapists who successfully help people with severe anger issues, but since her sincere suggestion to a man who flew into a maniacal, off-the-charts, scalding rage was turned down, walking away from the relationship was her healthiest choice. Or, as Francie said, "it was my only choice."

27

Your First Date In Years

Don't ask. Don't tell. Don't lie. That's your mantra, your Vedic hymn, and your hallelujah chorale, and don't you forget it.

Can you actually figure out numerically in days, months, or years how long it's been since you had a date with a new person? This is not about meeting someone casually at a party or chatting with someone you work with; it's a whole different scene. This is your first date since you've been on your own again. This is a date with someone you are attracted to who asked if you'd like to have dinner next Friday … the day is set. At seven o'clock your date will pick you up to go to the Courtyard Cafe … the time and place are set. Then the jitters begin. And the *what ifs*:

What if he tries to move too fast? What if he expects the date to end up in bed? I know that sex is a lot more casual nowadays, but will I be able to be intimate with another man after twenty-nine years with my darling husband? How will I feel about it later if I am?

Try not to spoil the evening before it even happens. You're in your late sixties and perfectly capable of deciding for yourself how you want your evening to end. It's entirely up to you. You might make your own decision in advance of the evening: definitely no sex on a first date, and maybe not for many dates. If, and I only say *if*, you decide to change your mind the night of the date, you don't instantly become a wanton trollop. The point is you alone have control of your actions; whatever you want is what you should do, and no one else gets to decide what you do or do not do with your body. Once you're clear on that, you're good to go.

The day is here. He picks you up, and you go directly to the restaurant where he's reserved a table for two in the no-smoking section. The room is filled with good-looking couples and groups obviously enjoying their evening, and you are bursting to find out more about your date. Stop right now. Look again at the top of the chapter: Don't ask. Don't tell. Don't lie. The same caution applies to both men and women.

A date, especially a first one, is not the time for a quiz. A new man or woman in your life is neither interested in a barrage of personal questions nor in more information than he or she wants to know about you. When you ask too many questions or reveal too much of yourself, it sends most people in search of a less intense, more mysterious companion.

The choice of a common interest is good to pursue: "Do you like to read fiction or nonfiction?" If reading is a common passion, then you've struck a nice note with that opener. Or, "Last night I saw a rerun of *Key Largo*; the story stands up today even though it was filmed in the fifties. Do you like old black-and-white movies?" A little bit of yourself is fine: "I just got back from a family gathering in Vermont. There were seventeen of us. Are you from a large family?"

Do not go anywhere near the following topics:

> Was it you who wanted the divorce? What went wrong in your relationship, and are you looking to remarry anytime soon?
>
> Don't ask about his psychic dreams, and absolutely shut up about your karma and aura.
>
> Don't give out finicky details of your weird diet or despair aloud that there isn't one thing on the menu in front of you that you can eat without breaking out in red blisters.
>
> Don't ask if he's updated his will since his wife walked out.
>
> Don't discuss your finances or ask about your date's insurance policy.

Don't mention that your senile father lives with you and that he likes to shoplift.

Don't pressure your date with sexual innuendo, implying you're a hot number.

If you insist on questioning your companion's personal life or loading your date with explicit and unasked-for details of your own difficulties and eccentricities, then you can safely count on this being your first and your last date, at least with this particular person. Your sins may have been scarlet, but don't load a new person with your past crimes. It's smart to tell the truth; it's also wise to not tell all of your past truths to a new person. So when you feel the urge to turn state's evidence on your entire life, opt instead for a huge, gooey, decidedly viscous dessert ... at least it will keep your mouth busy.

28

The Angry Adult Child You Could Inherit

For over a year you've been deeply involved with a wonderful new romance that's becoming more serious by the hour, and you're both over the moon with happiness. The two of you can hardly bear to be apart. He's funny, you're funny, everything either of you says is riveting, and as a team you possess insight into each other's feelings that is both thrilling and comforting. Finding love this late in life is an unexpected joy for both of you. Overall, life is sweet. However, there is one stubborn hitch that's not going to go away until you face it.

His oldest daughter is convinced that her parents never should have divorced and that they will likely get back together if you disappear. She's decided that you are the thief, the varlet who is spoiling her life, and no one will take her mother's place in her dad's life if she can possibly prevent it. She's made it obvious from your first meeting that she hasn't even the slightest preparedness to try to like you, and she makes no attempt whatsoever at surface politics.

Well, here you have it—the first real challenge since you met your jewel of a man who you have every reason to believe will remain solidly by your side in the years to come.

In a divorce situation, healthy, mature children almost always handle a new parental relationship better than immature children who, without cause, will disapprove of practically any new choice. But how do you handle an adult child who hates your presence in her father's life? It's hard not to take it personally, not to let it interfere in your happiness, yet you stand to lose your chance for a beautiful future unless you find a solution fast.

The first thing you want to do is talk about it openly with her father when you have him alone. Ask him if there is any truth to what the girl said, or if it was just wishful thinking on her part that there ever was a possibility that he and his wife might reconcile.

It's important to show him that you understand his daughter's loyalty to her mother as well as her disappointment over her parents' divorce—no father wants to have his grown daughter seen in a poor light.

If there is no thought of reuniting with his ex-wife, you can ask him to speak to his daughter so that she understands fully that his life, and whom he chooses to spend it with, is not her responsibility. It's important that he understand that you don't intend to either ignore her attitude or put up with it.

It's not exactly news that most men can handle confrontation with confidence on a professional level, but they're often pathetically hopeless at confrontation on a personal level. He'll probably try to avoid it and suggest that it will all go away once she gets to know you better and sees how great you are. Unsatisfactory as his response may seem to you, it shouldn't be a big surprise. All he wants is peace without emotional face-offs.

But ask him if that's how he solves thorny business situations when they arise, at which point you can expect a little mumbling on his part. Then, he'll probably switch lanes abruptly and suggest an early movie or ask what happened at the dentist this afternoon, as if anything ever happens at the dentist that doesn't hurt or that you're dying to relate.

In other words, he really doesn't want more talk about you and his daughter and he wishes you'd drop the conversation forthwith.

You can argue, get mad, or yell at him, but it will have as much effect as kicking a wet log. The problem is in your court, and if you want to get this matter out in the open, you will have to handle it yourself. Once that decision is made, you realize that the only effective way to express your true feelings on the issue is in a direct manner.

Rest assured that if it wasn't you, if it was any other woman in her father's life, (are you listening? *Any* other woman), that she, too, would be as well loved by his daughter as a dead mouse in her porridge. Your confrontation must be face to face—a phone call is a chicken way to do it. Try to fix a date in her lunch hour or for an early breakfast meeting.

She'll probably be uneasy to see you alone, so make it as short and simple as possible for her. You might tell her, "I'm sorry that your father's relationship with me is a threat to your comfort, and I can very well understand that, for you, it would have been nicer if your father's reality had paralleled your fantasy. But I want to make it clear (all this in a friendly, matter-of-fact way) that I'm not going to try to convince you I'm an okay person or devote time to getting you to change your feelings about me."

She'll probably start to relax when you explain further, "I don't need to have you like me. Maybe it will happen over time, or maybe not, but for now, I ask and expect that both of us be polite and civil to one another. How about we both give it a try? I know I'd like to do that."

Once she realizes that you're not forcing yourself into her life, things should improve. She'll be further relieved if she knows that you want her and her father to remain close and that you don't plan to be with them every time they want to get together. Then smile reassuringly, pay the tab, and get going.

She may not like you any better, but no doubt you'll at least gain her somewhat reluctant respect. Leave it for her to figure out that it's likely pointless to put her father through more hell over something that she's powerless to change.

Of course it's not just the new woman in a single father's life who can be a target for disapproval by his child. How about a son or daughter who gives strong signals of dislike towards their mother's new boyfriend?

Certainly it causes discomfort, and often argument, when children disapprove of their newly single parent's love interest, but sometimes your kids can size up a rotten choice quite accurately. Don't discount a warning too quickly; at the very least give it credence for protective concern on their part. Think about it. You'll be able to figure it out.

Your Healthy Attitude is Key: Part Three

29

Get Body Smart

What kind of shape are you in? It's okay—the door's closed, and no one's looking over your shoulder. Are you happy with that image in the mirror? Are you happy with your weight? How is your physical endurance? Are you sleeping well at night? Are you drinking too much? Smoking?

How long has it actually been since you paid serious attention to your own health? You were worried about your partner for so long that your own needs no doubt took a back seat. But now that you're on your own, it's high time you take better care of yourself. You're much too valuable a person to not give yourself the same care and attention you'd give your best friend. There's a host of things that affect health positively. Sensible diet, vitamins, daily exercise, and good sleep patterns all contribute to fitness, self-esteem, clear thinking, and accomplishment.

If you're resolute about getting in better shape, the first thing to do is get a complete physical check-up with your family practitioner. Go for the works—every test known to man. And don't forget a colonoscopy and a bone scan and bone density check; these tests are especially important when you've logged a few years. Follow up your tests with any suggested visits to other specialists, and then talk frankly with your doctor once all the results are in.

A holistic doctor can put you on a sound program of whole food supplements and vitamins; most medical doctors know zip in this particular area. Actually, if you're looking for a new doctor, you can probably find one who is a qualified MD with extended training in holistic alternative treatments, allowing you the option of both medical approaches. I'll never forget my first experience with holistic medicine: the first thing the doc suggested, when she reviewed my food preferences, was to stay away from animal fats and stick with *the no-legged fats*. Meaning olives, nuts, and fish oils.

If your doctor agrees, join a health club and go three times a week for yoga stretches or low-impact aerobic workouts. Consider swimming as a good choice to ease aches and stiffness. Or make a promise to yourself to walk every morning regardless of rain, sweltering heat, cold, or humidity. If you are willing to try something new, take on a newspaper route and you'll *have* to walk or bike to deliver the papers each morning. Within weeks, if it doesn't kill you before then, you'll start feeling stronger and livelier.

But even if you get totally ridiculous and exercise nonstop for eight hours a day, diet sternly, toss down a cartload of vitamins, and have undisturbed perfect sleep each night—it still won't recapture the body you had at twenty-two years. Perhaps the only way you'll get the body of a twenty-two-year-old is to buy him or her several drinks. Okay, okay, exceedingly bad joke. *However*, if you go regularly to a yoga group or a low-impact aerobics class, or stick to a fixed (it doesn't have to be vigorous) walking schedule, and follow a proper diet (i.e., skip desserts and heavy carbohydrates, get on a good vitamin regimen), you *can* feel and look your standout best. You'll feel so proud of yourself that it'll be worth every raw carrot and every missing potato chip. Obesity is never okay. Never, never, never.

Personally I like the idea of a buddy system for weight loss. Together, you and a friend can set goals and give one another a boost if you get discouraged. Working in tandem is part of the many success strategies from Weight Watchers. You don't *have* to lose pounds with someone else, but it's pretty nice to get and give support when needed.

If you're a heavy drinker and it concerns you, get to some AA open meetings and listen to what happens to people's lives when alcohol is allowed to take control. If you relate to any of their stories, you will know what to do: just keep going back.

If you take sleeping pills every night and you're afraid of becoming, or already are, dependent on them, perhaps you should talk with a doctor or call a drug help line (the number's in the front pages of your phone book), because there are better solutions to erratic sleep patterns. For example, exercising in the evening followed by a relaxing hot bath and lights out at ten thirty every night can work wonders. Don't crawl into bed, defeated, at two o'clock in the morning on one day, seven o'clock at night on another, and midnight on still another. Train your body to expect to sleep at ten thirty or eleven o'clock every night, and stick to it conscientiously until you're able to fall asleep naturally without sleep aids. Also helpful is using a good down, or water-filled pillow that supports you head, neck, and shoulders in the same alignment as if you were standing.

And then there's smoking. Oh yes. A lot of us still remember when it was considered debonair to smoke. Bogart and Bacal. The Marlboro man.

These days when I look at smokers, I see only *dumb*, especially on freezing-cold winter days when they're shivering outside an office building, but still puffing away. I see people who are smart in so many ways, but who refuse to take seriously a mass of negative information that reliably reports lung cancer, emphysema, heart disease, and underprivileged misery caused by smoking cigarettes. And it's not only the smokers who suffer and have to put up with dirty ashtrays, dirty looks, stinking breath, and polluted air—it's everyone else around them who doesn't smoke. Eventually, smokers will leave a lot of widows and widowers and sad children and grandchildren behind. But one sure benefit their survivors will enjoy is the knowledge that they no longer have to breathe second-hand smoke.

What about your eating habits? How about your food choices? Are you neglecting a proper diet? A good move is to set up an appointment with a nutritionist if your eating pattern is screwy. The right foods (right for you, that is) can regulate your mood, your body weight, and your energy level. If you're too thin, a recommended diet will take you off the scrawny list. "You can never be too rich or too thin" may have gotten Wallis Simpson what she wanted, but unless you want to marry a boring, cheapskate, Nazi-leaning dethroned king, it's hokum advice. Too thin is perhaps the most un-feminine way for any older woman to look; curves triumph over stick figures any day. A mature woman is better advised to keep flesh on her face and forfeit her fanny. Ditto for an older man. Both men and women over sixty look older than they are when they're too thin. Slim, however, isn't too thin. Nor is lean or slender too thin; it's just skeletal that's too thin. Runway models for years have been impossibly thin (size two or four—much, much thinner than the average woman), but recently a major fashion house in Spain announced it will no longer employ models thinner than a European size forty, the equivalent of an American size eight. The change was prompted by concern over the rising number of Spanish women suffering from anorexia in their efforts to compete with rattle-boned models. Let's hear it for that Spanish designer!

If you're too heavy, a proper nutritionally balanced diet along with regular exercise will let you drop unwanted pounds. Nutritionists and diet counselors are listed in the yellow pages of your phone book. Everything will improve when you eat the best foods in sensible quantities. Not only will your shape benefit, but so will your skin, nails, hair, and outlook. You'll feel more positive and look fabulous. Your weight is your own responsibility, but most fat people are heavy because they stopped caring at some point; gradually it got out of hand. We're all victims of habits, bad and good. Perhaps cooking classes and magazine articles may lead you to the right foods. Experiment. Learn. Be a beginner once more because nothing happens until you decide to make it happen.

Yoohoo! It's a brand new world out there. Tougher. Not so forgiving. For the first time in many years you're on your own again. You can mope, and no one will want to be around you, or you can embrace your new situation and love the results of reshaping your life. When you consider the alternative, what can you lose? Guilt? Weariness? Extra pounds? Sore back? Depression?

You decide.

30

Perking Up Brain Activity

Can you complete the *New York Times* Sunday crossword in an hour without outside help? If so, you can just turn the page right now, because you certainly don't need to read this bit of cheerleading. In fact, you're probably so darned quick you could get a job at the *Times* writing those puzzles! Did you ever try to write one?

For the rest of the crossword solvers who automatically turn to the medium-easy puzzle to solve, this is worth your time.

It's comfortable to work at a level where we have success, but does it keep the brain nimble? If you breeze through the medium-easy puzzles, then you might enjoy trying something that's more of a challenge; bump it up to the next level, whatever that next level is. At first it can slow you down somewhat and you could even end up with a few blank spots on the grid when you're done. Frustrating? Maybe. Seriously damaging to your ego? I doubt it. When you push yourself to a higher level in any intellectual pursuit, you'll find weaknesses to address. For example, if the new level of puzzle solving shows a lack of strong word comprehension, it could be that you need to raise your reading skills as well. It's all tied together. Age has nothing to do with it.

Lead researcher in the field of the aging brain, Mary N. Haan, MPH, Dr.PH., of the University of Michigan, told the attendees at The World Alzheimer's Congress 2000 in Washington, DC, "Cognitive decline doesn't have to be inevitable. Indeed mental tests given for ten years to almost six thousand older people found seventy percent maintained brainpower as they aged. Particularly protective of the brain is an increase in intellectual activity during adulthood."

Dr. Amir Soas of Case Western Reserve University Medical School in Cleveland advised, in the August 2000 issue of HEALL (Health Education Alliance for Life and Longevity publication), "Pull out the chessboard or Scrabble game. Learn a foreign language or a new hobby. Take up a musical instrument. Organize a bridge group. Do anything that stimulates the brain to concentrate."

"And read, read, read", he wrote, in an article on creating new brain cells, for a *Discovery Health Newsletter* in July 2007.

How do you rate yourself as a reader? If we place Harlequin Romances written in simple vocabulary at one end of the reading scale, and Russian novels with their complexities written in French at the other end (French being the language of the Russian literati), where would you place yourself? Think about it: if raising your reading level a notch exercises your brain, makes you more nimble mentally, and improves both your knowledge and vocabulary by raising awareness, it's bound to improve your life in general.

It doesn't mean you have to abandon your typically favorite type of novel or magazine in favor of something deeper or more difficult to read, no one volunteers easily to do that. The more complex reading would simply be additional reading. You can make room for new books or articles written with better language and thought-provoking ideas. The knowledge gained will stay with you for life. Dr. Soas continued, in his *Discovery for Health Newsletter* article, "It's a growing conclusion of research that fogged memory and slowed wit are not inevitable consequences of getting old and that reading tops the list of the steps people can take to protect their brains.

"And cut back on TV," he further insisted. "When you watch most television entertainment, your brain goes into neutral. Only a few years ago scientists believed the brain was wired for ever before age five, and that over the ensuing decades a person irrevocably lost neurons and crucial brain circuitry until eventually mental decline became noticeable.

"Not quite," Dr. Soas said. "Scientists now know the brain continually rewires and adapts itself; even in old age there's evidence of some new neuron growth. The two most important things to exercise a brain are mental activity and physical workouts. A healthy brain needs lots of oxygen pumped through healthy arteries."

An April 2007 televised debate, on the plasticity of the human brain, was anchored by award-winning Canadian journalist Steve Paikin, host and moderator of TVO's *The Agenda*. Among the noteworthy panel of psychiatrists and science writers, was clinical psychologist, professor Jordan Peterson from The University of Toronto (formerly at Harvard University), who made a spectacularly encouraging comment: "Fluid IQ, which we know tends to decline from the approximate age of thirty, can be reversed at age fifty by about fifteen years, simply by engaging in regular aerobic and strength-training exercise. And you get smarter, like you used to be. The brain is an organ after all and needs cardio-vascular exercise to remain healthy".

Wow! What an opportunity for us all, and the improvement costs zero dollars.

31

Two Quick No-Cook Soups

Almost nobody in their right mind would ever ask me for a recipe, but here are two dishes that pass every possible test for a non-cook. They can be prepared in a matter of minutes from start to finish. They are great tasting and nutritious, and there are only a couple of things to clean up afterward. They get my vote.

Green Soup

I choose eight (8) from the following list of raw green vegetables (the darker the green the better): parsley, broccoli, fresh peas, spinach, cucumber (with skin and seeds), unpeeled zucchini, lettuce, green beans, green pepper, kale, collard greens, asparagus and beet tops. You can think of more, and decide how much of each to use.

Wash and cut up vegetables, then puree in a blender. Room temperature or heated, pour immediately into soup bowls. I sprinkle the soup with sunflower seeds and serve it with rice cakes spread with wasabi, and a favorite creamed cheese.

Red Soup

I choose three (3) kinds of fresh organically grown red fruits from my favorite produce market plus one banana per person. My favorite combination is fresh raspberries, fresh strawberries, and fresh watermelon, with banana and pure cranberry juice (or orange juice) till I get the right consistency. I like it pretty thick. Serve chilled or at room temperature with fresh cornbread. It's truly a versatile concoction; some days I call this soup dessert and serve it with grated coconut and a fig bar.

As a kid, I remember every meal that wasn't Kraft Dinner was made from the kind of meat that hardly ever came in one piece, usually minced hamburger. It came in various disguises as stew, meat loaf, croquettes, meat balls or patties. Add ketchup, potatoes, and a boiled-to-kill-all-vitamins soggy vegetable. Finish off the meal with rice pudding or Jell-O. I grew up on that diet, as did everyone I knew. If the day's veg were Brussels sprouts, then my brothers and I would first check out the dessert to see if it was worth gagging through those rotten little cabbages to get to the semi-good stuff.

Who would have thought I'd end up eating the kind of foods I do today and loving it? If you'd told me when I was a youngster that broiled portabella mushroom caps stuffed with creamed goat cheese and topped with raw honey and pine nuts were what I could look forward to, I probably would have hitchhiked straight out of town. But for sure not by way of Ethiopia, which is where we were told that all those kids lived who were hungry for want of Brussels sprouts. And if they were eating something even worse than Brussels sprouts, which just is not possible, it's a country I would never have taken my chances on.

According to the University of California–Berkeley, the ten top nutrition stars are broccoli, kale, cantaloupe, carrots, mangoes, pumpkins, red bell peppers, spinach, sweet potatoes, and strawberries.

In general, don't worry about making a list, just look for fruits and vegetables with the deepest pigments for the highest antioxidant counts.

The following is a list of healthy, high-energy brain foods:

- Seeds and nuts: try sprinkling poppy and sunflower seeds and millet on salads and enjoy plain, unsalted popcorn and Brazil nuts as snacks.

- Brown rice, lentils, black beans, pinto beans, lima beans, and split peas: add these to your favorite salads, soups, and entrees.
- Fresh fruit juices: for highest yield, select fruit that is heavy for its size.
- Fresh vegetable juices: you'll find weird combinations of vegetables that are fun to try in the cookbook section of any health food store.

Skim milk has fewer calories than whole milk. Fish and skinless turkey have fewer calories than beef and pork. And I choose green tea instead of coffee. Actually, this is an outright lie on my part; coffee's still winning, but I'm working on it.

32

Stress Got You?

Stress is possibly a problem for you right now. It's not something to dismiss lightly because it can and does make you miserable. In fact extreme stress can strip all joy. Being alone for the first time in years can produce a level of stress that hits you in almost every aspect of your life, adversely affecting your sleep at night and leaving you tense and upset during the day. Your eating habits, too, are probably off: you're not eating enough, or you're eating everything in sight.

If it goes on too long, or if you can't handle it, you would be wise to seek counseling to get you over the worst hurdles. There are also a number of ways you can significantly help yourself.

I've been there. And so have tons of men and women facing life on their own. First thing in the morning, before even getting out of bed, I begin with stretches. I lie flat on my bed and scrunch around until I'm positioned diagonally across the mattress, reach my arms way back over my head, and alternately flex and point my toes. Almost immediately I feel the kinks pull straight as I focus on one good thing in my life: one talent or ability, or one good memory of a kindness, or a new job prospect, or a lunch date next week with a friend. I take a deep breath through my nose to swell my belly to the count of four, hold that breath for five counts, and breathe out through my mouth to the count of six. I repeat the deep breathing exercise till I can actually feel the tension relax and leave my body.

Next, I sit on the side of the mattress and drop my head to one side to meet my shoulder and hold it, reverse the stretch to drop my head to meet the other shoulder and hold. I do this a few times. Now I turn my head slowly to look backwards over one shoulder, return to center, then rotate my head slowly to look over the other shoulder. Each time I do this stretch, I try to look further back until I can see the room behind me. This exercise not only helps reduce tension in my neck, it's a great one to help keep my neck limber so I can look properly over my shoulder when I back up my car. That's my little routine to get going each morning. You can decide what stretches are right for you to do before you get out of bed.

Once you're up and mobile, a tall glass of water will re-hydrate you after a night's sleep. For many people meditation is a helpful tool to reduce stress. Get into loose clothing. In a quiet room sit comfortably in a straight chair, feet flat on the floor, arms relaxed, and hands resting palms up on your thighs. You might want to close the curtains and turn off your phone. Understand that meditation takes practice; it will become easier as you continue on the path of stress reduction. Meditation is valuable time to empty your mind of all thought. In order to do that, you will concentrate on a single word or a humming sound such as "omm." Begin with deliberate deep breathing, and say the word "omm" as you let out each breath slowly through your mouth. Continue to focus on deep breathing and drawing out your word for the full length of the exhalation.

After fifteen or twenty minutes, you will feel calmer. Fresh fruit and a cup of decaffeinated green tea would be a nice way to follow your meditation. Try to steer clear of caffeine; it will only sabotage your hope to reduce stress.

Jean Carper, author of *Food: Your Miracle Medicine* lists caffeine, chocolate, cheese, alcohol, yeast-risen bakery goods, red wine, aspartame and MSG as foods most likely to trigger headaches. Since the object here is to lower your stress level, it makes perfect sense to cut out foods that may invite extra tension. Jean Carper also gives her readers a fountain of information on how to recognize food intolerances, which foods will reduce anxiety, plus proven ways to lower blood pressure.

Her writing is packed with fact and knowledge to promote better health through optimum food choices.

A huge stress factor for me was the state of my finances. I would wake in the night in a panic about money: Can I make it through the month? What if there's an unexpected expense to be met? My credit card balance is preposterous, and the rate of interest on my balance is in the stratosphere! I cannot believe how many months I went through that same routine every sleepless night before I took a stand. Three years of an interest rate of nineteen percent is what I'd been paying. I had to find a better solution.

I called my card carrier and told them I was thinking of moving to a new company because the interest rate they were charging me was atrocious. A friendly voice on the line said she thought they could do something for me. She passed me along to her supervisor, and inside four minutes—I swear that's all—four lousy minutes! I had relief. He asked, "How would you like to remain with us, with the same credit line, but at a 9.6 percent locked-in rate?" I almost fell off my chair. That was ten points lower than I'd been charged for all the years I'd been a member on their sucker list. Did I tell him I'd need a minute to think about it? No, I did not. I whooped yes, yes, yes! I may have given him a serious headache for his good news, but I really didn't much care; his company had been giving me a serious headache for years. An added note here: a few months later I wanted to make an unusual purchase at six thousand dollars for a used car and asked for a further drop in interest rate and was given a new *ongoing rate* of 7.9 percent.

My next step was obvious. Now that I had a break in my rate, I decided to double up my monthly payments and not use my card until I had a zero balance; if I didn't have enough cash for a purchase, I didn't buy it. This may sound like kindergarten stuff to anyone who's never had debt, but when money worries seem unsolvable, people sometimes act as though they can't do anything about it and, as a result, remain frozen by their debt. Having come out the other side of the nightmare, I can tell you it's the biggest reducer of stress you can imagine. To have no debt is to have peace of mind.

If you have access to the Internet, you can type in "free credit card counseling" or "credit solutions counseling" and let the computer search for and display the information. Some of the sites are geared toward businesses, but many are for individuals who want to learn how to pay down debt. Other sites give information on money management to help you budget your money and make it simple to actually plan to save some cash; these sites are available by typing in "free financial seminars," "free tax and financial planning," or "free financial planning seminars." Yes, the finance companies that sponsor these sites do hope to get your business, but they're not pushy, and it's made clear from the beginning you are under no obligation whatsoever. Many of them invite you to enjoy dinner as their guest at a free educational workshop. These sessions are usually very well attended. And the dinner? Well ... when it's free don't expect four-star dining, but you won't leave hungry, and you will learn useful tips you can easily apply to your own money management situation.

On one of her regular *Today Show* appearances, financial editor Jean Chatzky gave her percentages for sensible spending/saving habits:

- Fifty percent on must-haves: mortgages or rent, utilities, insurance, food etc. Clothes such as a winter coat and snow boots are must haves

- Twenty percent on savings: out of each monthly income check, put aside 20 percent in a separate bank account until it's enough to purchase a bond, a savings certificate, or a blue chip stock

- Ten percent on building your bank balance for a surprise hit or a rare expense: a new roof, the house needs painting exteriorly, a new car

- Twenty percent on wants (For these purchases use cash only!): a vacation, a night at the casino, restaurant dinners, new golf clubs, a bicycle, a faux-leopard coat

Jean Chatzky further cautions to record every single money transaction: every check you write, every deposit made to your account, every automatic withdrawal from your account, every ATM use. If you are a senior, you can ask your banker about forgivable monthly service charges and free traveler's checks.

Finally let's look at stress and smoking from a new angle. You know it, everybody knows it, no one needs another Do Not Smoke it's-rotten-for-your-health lecture, but have you looked at the high cost of smoking as a stress factor? A person who averages a carton of cigarettes a week will spend perhaps $80 (tax included) each seven-day period, depending where you live. Now multiply that figure by fifty-two weeks in a year, and the cost is in excess of $4,000 dollars annually. That's a nice, tidy sum.

Instead of letting that money do all sorts of disgusting things to your throat and lungs, think of it as "green energy," cash in the bank. When you smoke cigarettes, you light a match, and the cash goes up in smoke. You can find better ways to spend your money:

- Your savings can buy you a beautiful digital camera and a new computer.
- Perhaps you need some costly dentistry. You now have the cash.
- Set off on an adventure. You can get premium accommodations on a seven-night Royal Caribbean cruise from Fort Lauderdale to the Canary Islands for $1100, or for $1800, you can sail away to Tahiti.
- A five-day ocean voyage from Miami to Key West to Nassau, with a stateroom suite and meals and lavish entertainment included, will cost you under $1100 on Carnival Cruise Lines. From Montreal you can have three weeks in Tunisia, return airfare, and all meals, wine, and hotel accommodations included for $2000 in Canadian funds.

Please note that prices will fluctuate with the existing economy. For an idea of current pricing, go to Cruises.com. The site will give you sailing dates and rates from either coast of North America. Check the Web sites of your preferred cruise lines, as well. If you find something that piques your interest, you may book right away through the Web site. Or, if you prefer, you can ask your travel agent to handle the details for you.

For sure everything in this chapter will help to ease your stress, but perhaps the single-most effective stress-buster of all is a strong engagement with life through meaningful work.

33

Safety Inside Your Home

At a garage sale I held when I was about to move to a new house, I had two cooking pots and eleven pot lids laid out on a card table. Something's not right with those numbers. And if you want to know what's wrong with them it's that I burn holes in pots of food cooking unattended on the stove. How often, you ask? Too often.

I'll put leftover stew on the stove to reheat—always on a high setting, it seems—and leave the room to do one little job till it's finished heating. But mostly what's finished is another formerly fine pot with a new hole in its bottom. And I'm left with yet another unmated pot lid. To say that cooking isn't my main focus of interest would be an understatement.

A friend put me on the right path—to the hardware store—for a small wall-mounted fire extinguisher, and a kitchen timer with an extra loud buzzer that I can hear from other rooms. Big improvement. It is kind of novel to now have a pot to go with every lid I own! And then there's the bonus of a dinner unburned.

Also in regard to food and eating, I learned to do the Heimlich maneuver on myself. Mostly you learn to perform the maneuver on someone else if something gets stuck in the windpipe. It's a method of manual application of sudden upward pressure on the abdomen of a choking victim in order to force a foreign object from the windpipe. But what do you do when you live alone and the victim is you? Simply lean over the edge of a table, the edge of a kitchen counter, or a hard-backed wooden chair. Press your abdomen against the edge with a quick thrust. Or make a fist. Place your thumb below and between the juncture of your ribcage, just above your waist. Grasp your fist with your other hand, and press it into the abdomen with a quick upward thrust. Repeat this movement until the object blocking your airway is expelled.

I spoke to two policemen in my area for other tips on safety inside the home, and I'm passing their tips on to you:

1. Even when you're at home, keep ground-floor windows and doors locked.

2. Install chains and dead bolts on all doors and extra strong locks on windows near a fire escape. Unless your door is solid wood or metal, never leave your key in the deadbolt; it's too easy for some low-life to break the glass and reach inside to turn the key.

3. Don't leave a key under your doormat or in any obvious place nearby.

4. Leave lots of lights on when you go out for the evening. At night leave a porch light on, one with a covered light bulb, so that a thief can't easily unscrew it or break it without alerting a neighbor or passer-by. Spotlights that shine on both front and back doors from an upper story are the best deterrents. The same outside fixtures can be rigged to turn on or off when triggered by any activity within a fifteen-foot range of the door.

5. When you're off on a trip, you want to cancel regular deliveries of your newspaper and your mail, and ask a friend or neighbor to keep an eye on your house and check inside for burst pipes or broken panes. Most insurance companies won't pay damages if your home has been broken into when it's been unattended for several days in a row. You can check your own policy for particulars. When you return home, if a window or door is open, broken, or unlocked, don't go inside. Go elsewhere to a phone and call the police.

6. Keep a photographic record of your valuables, and keep jewelry and important papers in a safety deposit box or in a wall safe in your home. A decal on the actual safe indicating that all items are properly video-recorded is advisable (n.b. I've taken all this info directly from a police pamphlet issued by the NPD in Naples, Florida).

7. Install smoke detectors in every area of your home—basement and attic included. Test the batteries regularly, and replace them when they are weak. You can tell they're weak when it sounds as if you have a cricket loose in your house.

8. Always keep a phone beside your bed and a flashlight within reach.

9. A phone call to the office of the Council on Aging or Office of Senior Services will tell you when the next series of presentations are scheduled in your area on how to protect yourself from scams, dishonest telemarketing schemes, and con games.

The telephone is the weapon of choice for criminals who talk gullible people out of billions of dollars a year. Older men and women are key targets. The president of the National Association of Attorneys General in Washington, DC says, "A telephone is like an assault weapon in the hands of a con artist." The federally sponsored Telemarketing Fraud Working Group and both CARP and AARP's criminal justice services advise to never give out your credit card number or information about your bank account to anyone over the phone. Also beware of any caller who asks you to send money or buy anything sight unseen over the telephone.

If you know certain areas of your home are more vulnerable for break-ins than others, you can pay particular attention to see they're made safer. I live in a single-storied house and keep the front and back door key-locked from the inside at all times—day and night. People who know me well know that I don't like to have anyone drop by without a phone call first to check if it's convenient; therefore if there's an unexpected knock at my door, nine out of ten times it's someone I don't know. I'll ask what they want without opening the door. If it's someone who asks to use the phone because his or her car won't start, I'll get the number or name of a garage or towing service to contact and I will make the call. But under no circumstance will I admit a stranger into my house. Never. I'd tell them to wait in their car till help arrives, or if we were in the middle of a wild blizzard, and I had a garden shed, I'd let them wait there. I don't have a garden shed.

34

Street Smarts

Street walks in the city can be good fun when you feel safe and unthreatened. Ultimately it's your responsibility to do everything you can to ensure your own safety. This is even more important if you are walking at night.

When you're out walking alone, especially if it's dark, leave your purse or shoulder bag at home, avoid back streets and alleys, and stick to populated areas. If you want to pick up a pint of milk or the evening paper, tuck a couple of dollars in an inside pocket along with a whistle. It's also very smart to have a cell phone with you when you're alone, whether walking or in a car.

Actually, if I'm out walking at night, I carry a "screecher" (it looks like a hefty lipstick case), a device recommended by the police that you keep, along with your hand, in your jacket or skirt pocket. When you squeeze it, it lets out an unholy, penetratingly high-pitched sound that alerts anyone within a hundred yards that something very bad is going on that shouldn't be going on. You can't always depend on your voice as a reliable "screamer." In frightening situations, your voice may seize on you and nothing more than a whimper gets out.

A man should carry his wallet in a front pocket of his jacket or pants instead of in his hip pocket; any worthy pickpocket with experience can lift a man's wallet from behind without his victim's immediate knowledge.

If a thief or mugger is after your purse or tote bag, it's best to throw it at him. Then set off your "screamer" or pull out your whistle and blow hard. He may drop or toss your handbag in the process of trying to get away from you and the alarming noise you're creating.

If you're walking from a building to your car at night and are accosted by a mugger for your car keys, toss them under your car or under another car close by. This allows you a chance to run away when the mugger has to crawl under the car to retrieve the keys.

On the street be aware of darkened recessed doorways and always pay mind to people around you. If you're nervous about someone walking behind you or coming toward you, get out into the street to attract attention—it will put anyone who's up to no good on notice. Cross over to the other side of the street if it is better lit and has stores that are open.

Never use an outside ATM by yourself at night, even in a well-lit area. It's too easy for someone to come up from behind and order you to give him or her your money. That person can have a gun or a knife—you just never know for sure. With so many crazies around, why chance it?

Because of incidents of people being accosted at bus and tram stops in the evening, many of the bus lines have instructed their drivers, upon specific request, to drop a passenger as close to home as possible. Before you get off a bus, look carefully for anyone suspicious standing in the shadows at the bus stop; if someone makes you nervous, don't get off at your stop, even if it means staying on the bus for another complete circuit. And under no circumstance accept a ride to your house from a stranger waiting in a car at a bus stop. Not even if he or she looks perfectly all right, has a great smile, and it's raining so heavily a ride would be more than welcome. One of the things taught in any self-defense course is that dangerous strangers do not look weird and frightening; often, in fact, they look quite the opposite.

If you travel by yourself in a car, keep the windows closed and lock the doors before you start the motor, and check in the back seat before you get in the car. I saw a creepy TV play where a woman got into her car in the poorly lit parking garage of her lover's office building and was strangled by someone crouched low behind the driver's seat. What made it even creepier was that it was a woman strangler! In that particular driver's case, I think she should have stayed away from the strangler's husband. Oh well, too late now.

When traveling in your car, keep a cell phone charged and at hand, and never pick up a hitchhiker.

Probably the very best protection for anyone driving or walking alone is awareness. Be aware of your surroundings. Keep to well-lit and populated places. Leave your handbag or briefcase at home. Have your house or apartment key in your hand, but keep your hand in your pocket as you approach your front door.

A phone call to your local police station will tell you when and where courses on personal safety are being offered free of charge to the public. In addition, my daughter, Martha, who graciously took time to read this material in manuscript form, asked me to please add that friends are our most important safety precaution. We need to make those friends and companions top priority, because traveling alone in thinly populated areas, especially at night, is bad for anyone and everyone at any age. People need to buddy-up.

35

Thieves of Comfort: Anger, Arthritis, Adult Hearing Loss, and Sleeplessness

Let's start with the first comfort-robber: anger.

The price you pay for being severely angry can only be measured by how little interest you have for anything else. Your anger explodes into argument and ultimatum followed by severing of ties between family members or friends. Other times, your anger implodes and leaves you gunpowder-mad, seething inside with bitter feelings of wanting revenge for the hurt that you suffered. Either way you're in major trouble.

It will probably be more helpful to talk with a therapist who is trained to sort out the real from the unreal than to thrash it out with your best friend.

The danger of discussing a seriously sore point with your closest friend is that you will dramatize the truth to show how right you are and how wrong the other person is in the struggle at hand. And your friend, who sees you're in no mood for logic, will tend to agree with you; this is a Band-Aid. The cure will come by working through critical anger with a professional. And anyone who has the guts to seek professional help is to be congratulated.

Without help from a trained professional, an angry heart will have little chance to sustain a healthy new romantic attachment.

Dr. Cardwell C. Nuckols, Ph.D., an expert in behavioral medicine for over twenty years is the author, with Bill Chickering, of *Healing an*

Angry Heart. He writes, "Anger may be tearing apart your heart, leaving you dispirited and longing for a new life. Never delude yourself into thinking that you can make your history and your anger disappear. By striving to channel the energy in your anger into positive actions, you can begin to rid yourself of debilitating anger."

Dr. Nuckols's important book is available through your library or at your booksellers.

The second comfort-robber: arthritis. At its worst arthritis is hell. "It is the single leading cause of disability among all ages." That's an amazing statement made by Paul Caldron, DO (Doctor of Osteopathy), research clinician at The Arthritis Center in Phoenix. "You expect it in one form or another starting in the middle years, but arthritis is an equal-opportunity deployer of pain."

You've likely been told by your family doctor that there is no actual cure for arthritis. But there are things you can do to reduce pain and stress from the disease.

- **Lose weight.** Being overweight will intensify the pain of arthritis; if you can reduce your weight so that it falls within normal range for your height, it will ease stress on your knees, hips, and lower back and lessen pain.

- **Follow a healthy diet.** You can further the improvement by sticking to a vegetarian diet, and if you notice any pain within a day or two of consuming a certain food or drink (such as wheat, dairy products, or alcohol), simply strike the item off your grocery list. Act as your own diet police.

- **Exercise daily.** Light exercise and walking daily, depending on the severity of your arthritis, will build muscle and flexibility to lessen the effects of the disease on your body. Inactivity encourages stiffness and pain. "Motion is lotion" is a favorite phrase of Toronto chiropractor Dr. James Fung, a specialist in the treatment of sports injuries. Ask your doctor about weight lifting, low-impact aerobics, yoga, or swimming for your condition, and learn from your doctor when to treat pain with heat or cold.

My own arthritis was complicated by onset osteoporosis and scoliosis, which is now being treated effectively by Dr. Fung through specific exercises and spinal adjustments without medication, a chiropractic approach known as the Pettibon system. My daughter, Lucy, who, luckily for me, researches all manner of holistic medical practices, alerted me to Pettibon; it's helped enormously.

Anything you can do to help make life less stressful should get at least one chance. If you can measurably ease your discomfort, you won't feel as creaky. Once you lighten up, the idea of a fresh start with a new love will seem like a swell idea again.

The third comfort-robber: adult hearing loss. Of all the comfort robbers, a hearing loss perhaps has the most severe effect on intimacy. Since solid loving relations are built on good communication, when one partner loses the ability to communicate to any degree, the relationship suffers. Privacy is threatened if your partner has to holler at you to be heard. As well as being so personally frustrating, your relationships with friends and family are also jeopardized. The University of California–Berkley states that hearing loss makes social communication a chore for half of all men and a third of all women over sixty-five.

Not to hear clearly what is being said to you is at times an embarrassment. Eventually people stop addressing you altogether because either they find themselves yelling to be heard or they pick up on your exasperation and annoyance and make a choice to not talk with you at all. It hurts to be ignored. But trying to communicate with a hard-of-hearing person can be puzzling or just downright difficult.

It also hurts to have someone mouth words in an exaggerated simplistic way as though you are either stupid or a foreigner ill at ease with the language. However, you are certainly ill at ease, and since you can't hear distinctly when another person speaks, that person might as well talk in tongues.

This is no time for ego to surface over a handicap. You really do owe it to yourself to get your hearing checked by an expert in the field.

Ask yourself, "What is more important? The fact a hearing aid advertises a handicap and is a blow to my pride? Or a growing remoteness between my loved ones and me?"

In a book called *Missing Words* by daughter and mother duo Kay Thomset and Eve Nickerson, with medical information by Donald H. Holden, MD., Dr. Holden advises anyone with a hearing loss to consult an otolaryngologist or an otologist (ear, nose, and throat specialist), to have an examination of the ear and a hearing test. Both specialists have MD degrees plus postgraduate training to prepare them as experts in problems of the ear and hearing. Don't settle for less.

Dr. Holden goes on to say, "One of the most crippling fears a person with a hearing loss faces is insecurity which can be overcome with the use of hearing aids. However, do not take yourself off to a hearing aid dealer first."

If your doctor recommends a hearing aid, you'll need his written prescription as well as your hearing test results so the dealer can match the hearing device to your particular problem.

Once the problem is looked after, intimacy with your lover is happily restored. Your friends and family will shout with glee. And when they get to be impossibly loud, you can always shut the magic hearing aid off!

The fourth comfort-robber: sleep deprivation. Tiredness affects your ability to reason, to learn, and to remember. It's impossible to operate at optimal levels when you feel exhausted all the time. It's easy to know when you're not getting enough sleep—your walk and talk are slow, your posture is poor, your eyes have a droopy, spaced-out look, and you feel groggy and as depressed and cranky as if you slept by night on the air vent over a parking garage. You may not see yourself in this light, but others clearly do.

Not sleeping properly takes a terrible toll on an active life that lately has become no fun at all. There you are yawning through a fabulous dinner with your honey, and while she's getting madder and madder, your yawns get wider and wider. All the time you're wishing you were home alone, asleep in your own bed. But you're seriously asking for a shove in front of a bus if you nod off in the middle of a special surprise reading of her latest love poem, (actually even a lot of well-rested people experience severe symptoms of fatigue with poetry readings).

It's a known fact that a good night's sleep gets harder to come by as a person ages, but there are several things you can do to improve an obviously impossible situation. Before running down the list, however, consider your mattress. If it is more than ten years old, you're due for a new one. An old one is likely home to more mattress mites (and their secretions) than you want to know about; a quick low cost solution is a washable, waterproof mattress pad. If, however, you're about to invest in new bedding, there's a smart mattress on the market now that features a zippered top section that holds a washable replaceable insert in order to control mites as well as body ash deposits.

This "to-do" list should improve your sleep habits:

- Retrain your body clock to depend on meals at expected intervals.
- Arrange your timetable to do business-related things—paying bills, making phone calls, and running errands—in the morning.
- Michael V. Vitiello, PhD., an expert in age-related sleep disturbance, and associate director of The Sleep and Aging Research Project at the University of Washington in Seattle, writes of natural slumps in alertness for most elderly people in mid-afternoon. He reports that if you don't get a proper sleep at night, a nap of thirty to forty-five minutes after lunch can help your body recharge and leave you refreshed and more attentive to detail. Backed by formidable bodies of research studies, Dr. Vitiello cites three distinct lifestyle changes that work just as well as pharmacological treatments, plus they work for a lifetime: regularize your schedule, exercise frequently, and be aware of what you eat. The first most important step in regularizing your schedule is waking up at the same time every day. The sec-

ond step is going to bed at the same time. Vitiello has conducted a number of studies linking regular exercise to better sleep in older adults. Even moderate exercise, such as mall walking, improves sleep. And being aware of foods that affect a night's rest is an often-overlooked strategy: spicy and rich foods can both cause problems. He adds, "Alcohol may help you fall asleep, but so will a blow to the head!" In fact, when you're trying to regulate your sleep pattern, you'll do better without caffeine in the evening. Keep all liquid intake to a minimum after six o'clock so you don't have to get up often during the night.

- For a while before bedtime relax with music or a satisfying book. Sit in a chair rather than reading in bed. Your bed is for sex and sleep.

- A hot bath or shower immediately before you retire for the night will make you drowsy. Try to sleep in a quiet, dark room of cooler-than-normal temperature. If you don't fall asleep after fifteen minutes, get up and go into another room to read until you are good and sleepy.

If you think this all sounds like you're being punished or that you're over the hill and your life is one big drag, take heart and don't be discouraged; within a few weeks of sticking to your new routine, you'll be back on track and feeling more like your old self. And when you do feel rested and livelier, stick to the new habits to which your body has responded positively. Your whole outlook will improve. Believe you can overcome a problem, and you're halfway there.

36

Dating After a Mastectomy

It wasn't till years later that I realized how brave and special my mother was from the minute she found out she had breast cancer. She was only fifty years old and single, yet at the time her first thoughts were about her kids and how we'd react to her news. We were actually not kids at all; we were grown-ups with kids of our own. She was the one facing surgery, yet she was the amazing one trying to put our fears to rest and make *us* feel better!

Because she'd always been powerfully self-sufficient, it seemed quite normal to the family that she would sail through her operation, the radiation treatments, and her recovery, and never refer to her mastectomy except to say she wouldn't be entering any bathing beauty contests. Guts and self-confidence were her two greatest strengths. As soon as she had her doctor's go-ahead, she took off for Florida, and within five months she was dating the most sought after man in her large apartment complex. My mom and Paul had twenty-three wonderful, loving years together. After he was gone, she kept on going alone just like the battered bunny in the TV ads.

Since then I've known friends who've had a single or a double mastectomy. Some were married at the time. Later some of those same women became widows or divorcees, and when they were ready to look for another partner, they were especially nervous and shy about beginning an intimate relationship with a new mate.

Perhaps this is you: You've been seeing a new man for a few months. He knows you've had a mastectomy because you've discussed it with him, but his knowing something intellectually is not the same as seeing you for the first time without a breast or without two breasts. Are you worried your new man will be repulsed by the scar tissue, consider you some kind of a freak? Or will he hold you close and admire your courage? Ultimately it's how you feel about your own nakedness that's the most important issue here. I understand very few women have my mother's self-confidence. But give men a break, please. We're talking about real men, not jerks.

Barbara Delinsky, one of the country's most popular novelists, has written a best-selling, must-have book titled *UPLIFT: Secrets from the Sisterhood of Breast Cancer Survivors*. Every woman who has been diagnosed with breast cancer should read her book. Consider it part of a vast support system that's out there for breast cancer survivors and their friends and families. In it she addresses the many concerns you might have about the disease from the moment of your diagnosis. Delinsky also addresses how various men and women handled intimacy after mastectomies. It's heartening to read testimonies from husbands and lovers who, while very concerned about both the cancer and the prognosis, never cared more about how his woman looked than he cared about her well-being.

All the men who contributed their thoughts in the book *UPLIFT* were warmly protective of their women. To a man, the main consideration was to assure the women they loved that breasts—one breast, two breasts, no breasts—were nothing compared to the whole woman. Each and every man wanted the woman he loved to be with him for the rest of his life. As one very smart man wrote: "A woman's life is so much more than the quantity and positioning of a little bit, or even a lot of flesh. Breasts don't laugh or smile or share brilliance or give kindness. Life is the true treasure; otherwise we'd save the breast and discard the woman. A living woman is beautiful, a dead woman isn't nearly so attractive." Barbara Delinsky gives all breast cancer survivors a gift of high hope and positivity with her book, *UPLIFT*.

37

To Share a Bedroom or Not

Big decision in your life? Another marriage, and before you move in together, you're wondering whether to start off with shared space or separate bedrooms.

Don't think I'd have to spend much time figuring out this one. For most older-yet-new couples there's only one no-hassles answer: two bedrooms with visiting privileges for special intimate times (even when those are every day).

Intimacy is a whole raft of shared moments not determined alone by sexual activity. It's snuggling up to watch a TV program, lying in bed reading or having an important serious discussion, a laugh, or a cozy afternoon nap. But for a restorative full night's sleep, there's nothing like your own bed in your own room, if possible. In a one-bedroom apartment, it's simply not an option, but maybe two double beds in the one bedroom is a solution.

Two bedrooms for actual sleep is perhaps the happier choice if you have the luxury of a second room. Most likely at least one of you snores. I've actually woken myself up snoring even though I would've sworn, and did swear, I was a perfectly quiet ladylike sleeper till I woke one night terrified by what sounded like a full orchestra tuning up their trombones, and whatever else, on my very own Sealy Posturpedic. That's a hard one to explain away.

A restless sleeper is kept awake by another person's night noises. And most probably each of you is up during a long night with a couple of trips to the bathroom. Maybe one of you needs less sleep than the other or handles insomnia by turning on the light and reading for an hour at some point during a wakeful night.

For a lot of people, especially women (and men who hate being nagged to hang up wet towels or leave the toilet seat down), having a bathroom of one's own is far more important than a separate bedroom. However, both bedrooms and bathrooms will take some negotiating to come as near as possible to what you want ideally.

To tip the scale toward two bedrooms versus a shared space, visiting back and forth can lend an air of fresh fun and surprise, undeniably an intriguing way to remain a little mysterious to your sweetheart. You can send your love red roses for no reason, and see if that doesn't get you a delighted night visitor.

And I know (from experience) that a full-scale mariachi band serenading him under his bedroom window at three o'clock in the morning will definitely get his attention—no doubt about it, but it may also have him thinking about locking you up in a secure psychiatric facility.

Perfecting your Hidden Skills: Part Four

38

The Fear Factors

Can you identify your biggest fear? Specificity is important here. It's not enough to say, "I'm afraid of what the future holds for me."

To identify money as a fear, for example, is *still* too unspecific.

The specific fear is: I'm worried that I might outlast my savings. So let's look at that one.

Concrete personal financial advice is what you need. You can start with your bank manager (who doesn't charge a fee), for some guidance. If your situation is complicated and still unclear to you after you meet with your bank manager, he can offer sound, conservative direction to a reputable financial planner to address your present and future positions. And your lawyer possibly has details of your spouse's will, or details of a divorce settlement regarding monies in your favor; a lawyer can also steer you toward a trusted financial planner.

Also you might decide to take an investment course to learn more about money. Watch your newspapers for upcoming speakers in your area who are scheduled to lecture on finance. Even if you already work with a financial consultant, it's smart to be able to keep up with him or her and be your own investment watchdog. After all, no one will care more than you whether your savings are growing at a reasonable rate. Financial courses usually appeal to solid men and women; this is another likely place to meet a serious partner. Smart people like smart friends.

Loneliness is another fear for many single-again adults. This, again, is too vague and needs to be broken down to specifics.

The specific fear is: I'm alone and uncomfortable leading a single's life. I didn't ask for it, and I dread the idea of facing who knows how many years of living alone with no one to love and care for.

The starting place is to find personal happiness through meaningful work, work that is mutually beneficial to you and a group that needs you, where something you do makes a real difference in other people's lives. The math is odd on this one: the more you give of yourself, the more you receive. And you do have a lot to give.

What sounds like an impossible equation is equally impossible to beat, because when you give of yourself in a meaningful manner, you attract people who will want to be close to you. Believe it; you won't be alone for long.

It doesn't matter if you are a man or woman, old or middle-aged, drop-dead gorgeous or plain as plain can be; there's something magnetic about genuine generosity and strength of character. Eleanor Roosevelt was no beauty queen, but her sincerity as a lecturer and newspaper columnist in her fight for social betterment won over a host of respectful followers. Winston Churchill was a dead ringer for a British bulldog, yet his strength and charisma brought England through a war; he stood up to the Nazis and earned worldwide admiration. I realize you won't be operating on a global level, but when you get involved in any worthwhile community project, you will find great friends among your co-workers.

"I'm a sixty-nine year old man; my wife and I used to have a busy social life with other couples back home." What are the specifics?

The specific fear is: When I retired, my wife and I moved to Florida and away from our old friends in Utah. My wife died quite suddenly shortly after we settled into our new condo five months ago, and I don't know anybody in the area.

Why not begin getting to know your neighbors by becoming active on your condo committee? It's kind of a thankless, tedious job in many ways, yet it will give you proximity to your entire condo community. Perhaps you have a useful skill to offer in accounting, decision-making, or personnel work that is needed on the committee? Oftentimes simply being a willing helper is requirement enough. After all there's no money in it, so you can be pretty sure that your offer to help will be welcomed.

It starts with finding one friend in the building complex, after which the ripple effect goes into play: perhaps your new friend is a widower, same as you, but the difference is he has a lady friend. Then you find out that his lady friend knows a few unattached ladies who want to meet suitable men.

A good relationship is perfect for your health; finding a special someone requires maturity and the basic preparedness to give and to enjoy being on the receiving end of companionship, support, and tenderness. It may take several tries before you find the right woman, but as long as you deal fairly with each woman, you will end up with a number of new friends.

Get out to all the neighborhood events—parades, ball games, soccer games, lectures, and art fairs—and talk to everyone around you on these occasions. Drink your morning coffee regularly at a busy local café where interesting people gather, and say hello to a person at the next table. Get involved with cancer walks and other fund-raisers that support causes you believe in. And look fresh and well put together whenever you go out of the house—that's for both men and women. You never know when and where you will run across someone who is going to be a special person in your life, so you want to look great every time you put your nose outside your door.

39

Stand Up for Yourself

Standing up for oneself is an acquired skill that, for some, doesn't come easily; yet without that skill you are a victim waiting to happen. Remember when your neighbor wanted to borrow your hall chairs for a PTA meeting, yet it took another two weeks to get them back, because her family came for a visit and she decided she needed to keep your chairs until they left town? It certainly didn't bother her that your hall looked naked in the meantime, but you said nothing; you didn't object.

How about when your son expects you to baby-sit his three sheep dogs whenever he feels like taking off for the weekend? Or when he expects to use your car any old time he wants? And what about your sister's outrageous request that, since you are alone and just rattling around your big house, you put up six out-of-town guests for her daughter's second wedding—people you don't even know and will never see again? Nervy? For sure, and one can only wonder why it is you keep meeting everyone else's needs before your own.

In small things it mostly doesn't matter, such as arguing a choice of a restaurant or one movie over another. In bigger things it matters plenty; there's something impeccably boring about a totally accommodating man or woman who allows, even invites, others to take advantage of his or her time, talent, or sweet nature.

If you're forever willing and available to fulfill the bidding of a demanding parent, an adult son or daughter, a spoiled grandchild, a needy friend, then of course you're allowed to sigh and smile bravely and assure everyone that you really don't mind. To which the general unspoken reaction, I wager, is, "Wow, what a sucker!"

You could hand out printed cards: *I am a martyr—walk all over me.* And even though a martyr can always extract a guilt-giving fee for being used unfairly, is it enough to compensate for your loss of self? It doesn't make you admired or more beloved; love has nothing to do with it. And surely recipients of your indulgence see you as a bit of a fool if you too eagerly put their needs before your own and rarely get to live your own life or have energy and time for your own plans. When you place so little value on your own time, finances, property, or abilities, you're bound to suffer some loss of respect from the very person receiving favor. It shouldn't surprise you. Users often ridicule people who help by sneeringly calling them "do-gooders."

Did you let yourself be coerced into taking daily care of one of your children's children? Even if your child needs your help until his or her financial picture is better, you should place a time limit on your agreement to take on the responsibilities of those kids and make everyone involved aware of those limits. You should never allow your goodness to be abused.

To be able to say, "You had these kids. You look after them," makes your adult child a stronger mother or father. It also makes you a more respected grandmother or grandfather and a better friend. But don't expect that reaction initially from a selfish grown child who still is, and always will be, your kid who expects you to be delighted to look after his or her needs. Especially if it's all he or she has ever known.

But listen: no one else is going to do it for you, so any time you resent a tougher person who exploits you, you have to stand up for yourself. Every time you don't do it, you become less and less of an authentic person.

If you take a chance and say in a calm voice, "I really don't want to do what you just asked me to do because I have other plans," then you become a believable human being who commands respect and appropriate consideration.

I remember a TV talk show I once watched on the subject of bullies and how they got to be that way. Two bright young men in medical school told how they had interned in a nursing home for a few months, and how some patients, so pathetically eager to please the attendants, brought out the darker side of each of their personalities. They found, to their horror, that they became verbally abusive of those patients who didn't expect courtesy or respect.

There they were: two decent young men with no histories of oppression or intimidation, honor students who were about to become doctors, yet they both admitted to verbal abuse because the frail old people in their care wouldn't make their needs known or object to increasingly rude and inconsiderate treatment.

It's a sad fact that when a person loses healthy aggression or the dignity to expect consideration, his or her personality is diminished and others will take advantage.

If you're in this situation, you're not alone. It still doesn't make it okay, and it will never be so until you can resist anyone who expects more of you than you feel entirely wonderful about giving to that person.

The bonus of daring to confront anyone who you allowed to intimidate you in the past is that you regain credibility. More likely the most exciting bonus is the look of utter astonishment on the face of someone who's always put his or her needs before yours when you stand tall and say, "No way. Not this time, pussycat. I have plans of my own."

40

Take Good Care of Friendship

A close friend is one of life's greatest gifts: a special person you like enormously and feel totally comfortable with, someone you find interesting and trust entirely with your secrets and fears. At times you can both laugh like hyenas or listen quietly to problems. You get together whenever you can, and you stay current with frequent contact by phone, fax, e-mail, blackberries, photos and letters. You appreciate each other's thinking, humor, and support. You're careful to never undermine your friend's self-confidence or act in a hurtful way. And you never, never divulge a confidence. You each value the friendship, applaud one another's achievements, and make sure to be there in discouraging times.

A friend will often outlast a love affair or a marriage if you treat your friend's feelings with care and respect and still continue to include him or her in your life when you're involved in a heady romance. However, if you're neglectful and put your friend to one side when a new romantic figure arrives on the scene, eventually the friendship reaches its limits of endurance, and only a fool or an egomaniac would ever let that happen.

41

A Man Finds His Lost Love

You've thought about her from time to time over the years. No, not every day. You had a busy life centered in your family and career, but at times when you felt discouraged or unappreciated, she would come to mind—the girl you couldn't forget. What ever happened to her? Where is she now?

When John Ludlow's wife passed away, he found himself single for the first time in over forty years. Last night when he put his pocket change on the dresser, he stared at the small gold monkey his once-upon-a-time girlfriend gave him in high school as a good luck charm. He's carried the trinket among his coins his entire adult life.

The next morning in his office, John told his son, "I want to find an old girlfriend."

"You're kidding?" was his son's quick response, till he saw his dad's serious face. "No, you're not kidding. Wow, she must have been someone special if she's still in your thoughts."

"Her name is Alice." John Ludlow motioned for Eric to close his office door and take the chair on the other side of his impressive mahogany desk, and he began.

Some twenty minutes later he smiled at Eric's disbelief, "And that's why I have to find her. I don't even know where she's living, but I am going to find her."

"Dad, I'm not sure how to say this, but you don't even know *if* she's living, do you?"

John heard the concern in his son's voice. "Not once have I ever thought she might not be alive—I think I would have known immediately if she'd died."

"What's amazing to me is that you still feel so strongly connected that you can't believe she might have died without your knowing it. Is it because you never got over her? And what about Mom, did you love her at all? She was very beautiful."

"She was difficult."

"She was difficult; I agree."

"When I met your mother, I was twenty years old, in my second year of med school on a student loan, and working part-time in construction to finance it. And when she told me she was pregnant, I dropped out of school to hire on as a full-time construction worker. It was her plan to marry a doctor, not a carpenter, so she was already feeling gypped when she married me. Then quite a few years later, after I started my own construction company, I got to wear a suit and have a nice office and make a lot more money than any doctor. However I still wasn't a doctor, and she still wasn't happy."

"Did you ever regret it? Marrying her?"

"And miss out on having you for a son, oh, no. No. I will always and forever be in her debt for that."

"Dad, let's say you do find Alice, but what if she doesn't want to see you? After all you wrote her 365 bloody letters, and she didn't answer one of them."

John started laughing, "It's worse than that: it was a leap-year, so I sent 366! I'd decided I would write her every day for a year, and if I heard nothing from her in that time, I would quit writing. As soon as we got to San Diego I mailed a letter every day from the post office. Maybe she never got them. Her mother could have grabbed them before they got to Alice. I think her mother interfered—kept my letters secret and left Alice in the dark about my phone calls."

"Could that have happened?"

"If you knew a Southern woman you'd get it right away: no scandal concerning her family is allowed to air. The disappearance of a daughter's boyfriend is considered scandal. The telephone operator told me each time I called that Alice wasn't home."

"You mean whoever answered the phone told the operator to say that?"

"For sure. Later the operator was instructed to say that Alice wouldn't speak with me and to please stop calling. After a month the number was changed to an unlisted one. At seventeen, both Alice and I were naive. I can only guess what she was told about me. But back then I eventually came to believe she really didn't want to hear my voice; anyway, I was afraid she'd hang up on me, so I just kept writing letters."

"Okay. So where does that leave us? I mean, I'm with you all the way on this one, and I guess the best place to start is the place you last knew her. That means going back to Tennessee."

"That means starting the search in Tennessee, you're right, but we don't have to go there physically. There might be an alumni association at our old high school. I can do that one by phone. There's also the Chattanooga newspaper morgue, but that would involve a visit or maybe hiring someone locally to research old microforms for weddings and births of babies. If she got married in Chattanooga, we'd have her married name to go by."

"If we had her married name, we could go after information year by year on an indictable crime or on anything newsworthy such as a robbery or an award ceremony. Or we could run a business search on her husband—see if he worked for himself or was ever promoted within a corporation. Maybe the guy got killed in a car accident or something, that'd be good, too."

"Not for him."

"Yeah, well, not for him."

"Listen, Eric, it means a lot to me to have your support on this. I guess you also want to see what she's like, see if I was totally wet about how strong things were between us. But the search may lead to finding her happily married to a perfectly great guy."

"No. That's not going to happen. We are going to find her. And she's going to be four hundred pounds and she'll crash through the airport barrier and lunge toward you with all this blubber floating behind her, and you, Dad, are going to want to hightail it for the hills."

"Come on, you crazy kid, let's get a quick lunch then see how much headway we can make this afternoon. I propose we try it on our own for ten days or until we exhaust our possibilities, whichever comes first. And if we run into a dead end, we'll go the professional people-locator route. What do you say?"

"That's good by me. I like the idea of doing it by ourselves, but not pushing it to the point of stupidity."

Ten minutes after they got back from the diner on the corner, John reported that there was no official alumni association at Mount Cedar High, only a committee appointed every ten years for reunion gatherings. The school's principal had informed him that the next reunion was five years off. "So that one's a dead end. But I'm remembering something about a book that was published not long ago about finding people you've lost track of. I'm going to try the reference desk at the library next, see if anyone there knows a title or the author."

"Okay, you go, and I'm getting on the computer here in the office to see what I can find. Going to run some search phrases for locating people. I've got to pick up your granddaughter from day care at two thirty, so I may be gone when you get back."

Inside an hour John was back in the office. He'd found the title of the book that he wanted in the library system, but it wasn't available at the local library. However, he did find something else at the bookseller's in the mall: *When in Doubt Check Him Out* by Joseph J. Culligan. Its subject is actually a woman's survival guide to prevent getting mixed up with a liar, a cheat, or worse, but, no matter, the ways of retrieving information would serve even if the reason for finding Alice was quite different. His son was still at the computer when he got back to his office.

"Hey, you're still here. This book is amazing; it's so clearly set out that it would be damn near impossible to hide from anyone who's seriously looking for you."

"Let's see it. Maybe we can follow some leads from the book, but use the computer to shortcut the search. I got a call from home that the sitter picked the baby up early, so she's already home. I've got extra time."

"Listen—there are twelve sections in the table of contents. Not all of them apply. We can eliminate tracing her through social security administration; she's sixty-two, my age exactly, so she's not old enough to be collecting social security benefits. Another unlikely one is through child support enforcement records. I'm dead certain we can eliminate that one. Ditto with bankruptcy records and abandoned property claims. That leaves only eight avenues of investigation."

"That sounds manageable. What's number one? Yeah, here we are: driving and automobile records. It says here to write to the Department of Motor Vehicles for the driving record of—and you name your person. Listen to this: The letter does wonders. You give the person's name and last known address, and a date of birth if you know it.' And you do know it, right, Dad? Of course, right," he grinned at his father's affirmative nod.

"I know it: January 9, same birth year as me."

"It goes on to say driving records may contain some or all of the following, and I quote, 'address, height, weight, hair color, eye color, social security number, date of birth, date of original application for a driver license. It will cover dates and locations of accidents. An accident report may include home address and phone number plus a name of an insurance company.' That's a lot of stuff."

"Also the author gives contact numbers for offices of driver licenses in each state. There are a ton of them for Tennessee, I'll choose one in

Nashville. Do you want to try this by phone, by fax, or by letter? Also it's likely all on the Net, if you want to go that route."

"Why don't I try a phone call, verify the address of their office, and find out how much the search costs so we can get that one started. And while I'm doing that, see what the book lists as the next approach."

"Okay, here we go—next are divorce, marriage, birth, and death records. You realize, even if she was divorced, we don't have a husband's name. Marriage records sound more likely, don't you agree?"

Fifteen minutes later John placed the receiver back on the hook, "I was able to do it all by phone! Can you believe it? They will fax the information to me within two hours: Alice's complete driving record; it will be charged to my Visa. It's kind of scary to think that anything on public record is available to anyone who asks for it. I don't think I would've had to even give my name if I were paying cash in person. How are you doing on the marriage records?"

Eric read aloud, "The book says 'If you do not know if your subject is married, you should ask for a search conducted for a span of several years.' Dad, for our purpose, is jurisdiction the same as county? Listen—it says you will need to contact each jurisdiction regarding the release of marital records. Some governments severely restrict the release of marriage records except to the bride and groom—that applies in New York City's five boroughs, whereas all areas in the State of Florida consider this to be a public record."

"New Yorkers are such pains in the ass at times. They also consider themselves more sophisticated than us hillbillies—can't understand why—so let's just assume that it's wide open in Tennessee. Does the book list county numbers? Anyway, that's not too serious. Chattanooga is in Hamilton County; I remember that."

"Actually there is an appendix of county mailing addresses in the back of the book, by state. Why don't you see how much you can do by phone again? Maybe they'll also fax the information and take your credit card. Dad, I've got to get going now. Liquor store, home, start the barbecue; the neighbors are doing a joint thing in the backyards tonight."

"Sounds like fun. I'll try for a ten-year span on marriage records. Talk to you in the morning."

♦ ♦ ♦

The next morning Eric was already in his dad's office making coffee when John arrived. John's face gave it all away; his smile was wide as a watermelon slice and his eyes were sparkling with life. "I spoke with Alice last night. How's that for a bombshell? Let me tell you what happened. First I was able to retrieve her marriage records. From that I got her husband's name."

"On a whim, late yesterday afternoon, I asked for a search of the National Cemetery System records through the Veterans Administration Department of Memorial Affairs, using her husband's name—I got that lead out of Culligan's book—and found he'd been an air force pilot. He died nine years ago from cancer, at fifty-three, in Memphis."

"And you phoned her? Good God, it's a wonder the woman didn't have an attack of some kind when she realized who was calling."

"'What took you so long?'—first words out of her mouth! I don't know if she realizes it," John laughed out loud, "but she said the exact same thing to me when I asked her to the senior prom forty-six years ago!"

Eric just shook his head in amusement at his dad's obvious happiness.

Later, John was still sitting at his desk cradling the mug of cold coffee that his son had handed him over an hour earlier as he recounted, word for word, last night's conversation with Alice. The part that had truly stunned John was when Alice told him she already knew where he was living and knew that he had a son. She even knew his address through records in the land registry office in San Diego and his phone number from the directories that are kept for major cities in all public libraries. She'd used a professional people-locator agency in Memphis to find him after her mother died, but discontinued the search when they reported he was living with his wife and child. John's heart had swelled to hear her say that she, too, hadn't forgotten.

He was strangely quiet at his desk, yet curiously his thoughts weren't about Alice or last night's extraordinary phone call. His unhappy deceased wife was the center of his reverie. He'd known her for six months before they married, during which time he saw her maybe once every couple of weeks. From their first date she was little else than a hectic woman in his bed. He knew so little about her when she told him she was pregnant, that when they later filled out the forms at city hall, most of her statistical information was news to him. Her middle name, her birth date and year, the fact she'd had a brief marriage previously annulled by her parents, even her home address were new facts of little or no interest. The marriage hadn't had a chance from the start, but in those days, if you got a girl pregnant you married her.

Psychiatrists, psychologists, and counselors had at various times diagnosed his wife as clinically depressed. And though they'd tried to assure John that a chemical imbalance aggravated by a giant ego had almost nothing to do with him, he knew he'd never loved the woman, had never even liked her very much. He was in medical school when they met, and she walked straight into the role of silent but fiercely willing sex partner. At the time, that's all he wanted. Even that wasn't to last.

As soon as Eric was born, his wife showed a complete lack of interest in her tiny baby or in her husband; it marked the beginning of psychiatric help that didn't work because neither he nor she gave the outcome enough priority. And every time John wanted to clear out, to ditch the marriage, it was the combination of guilt for never having loved her and the reality that he would almost certainly not be awarded custody of his son that prevented him from doing so.

When his son reached his teens, a new psychologist with a new approach effected a positive change in his wife that brought about a renewed interest in sex for her, but John was beyond caring, and her attempts at seduction ended in miserable functional failure on his part. A few awkward months later, their married life returned to limited conversations about facts, people, events, and schedules. Over the years there were women from time to time, usually on out-of-town business trips, but for the most part John had lived a life of forced celibacy.

Now John had a big worry. Alice was on her way to see John in ten days. He was excited beyond belief; the possibility of a loving reunion was on the horizon, but after such a miserable relationship with his wife he was worried. In fact, worried didn't begin to cover it—he was terrified that he would be a total flop if she wanted intimacy. Wouldn't that be the irony of his life? To want something forever, it seemed, only to fail when finally given the chance to be with the love of his life.

The phone at his elbow rang three times before his own-recorded message came on, then he sat without moving as Alice left information confirming her flight in a cheeky voice full of promise. When the line went dead, John dialed a number he didn't even know that he had memorized for the psychologist who had tried to help his wife years earlier. A secretary took his call, and within the hour the doctor called with news of a cancellation that would allow John an hour right after lunch.

John sat across the desk from the doctor fearing the worst, but the man was so straightforward and natural that within minutes John very clearly laid out his fears of chronic sexual dysfunction that went back to his troubled marriage. The doctor had treated John's wife and he knew of his former patient's death a year or so earlier. John told him about their son helping him find his long-lost sweetheart and about his own high hopes for her impending visit.

"We were separated right after high school by my parents' sudden decision to move across the country, and I can say truthfully that I've been missing Alice all my life. I really want to see her." The eagerness in his voice said it all. The doctor smiled in an understanding yet you-lucky-bastard-to-be-given-a-second-chance kind of a way.

"John, listen, I'm not going to go deeply into the difficulties that faced you and your wife; all that's behind you. She was a narcissist; her only interest in sex early on in your relationship was to have you admire her acrobatics. Your wife never had the capacity for loving—an exhibitionist is nothing more than an actress."

"The woman you've found again—Her name is Alice, you said? How do you know that Alice's husband wasn't impotent occasionally? The University of California–Berkley has publicized statistics stating that more than ten million American men are chronically impotent. The information and numbers cited were taken from reported cases, meaning patients seeking help from their doctors, but the true numbers that would include unreported cases are most certainly higher. Very definitely more men are seeking help since the advent of Viagra—and if you attach weight to the advertising copy from Pfizer, the pharmaceutical company that created Viagra, there are over forty million men occasionally or chronically in trouble in the United States alone."

"Do you think those figures are accurate?"

"Frankly, I don't think the actual numbers matter that much to any man that can't get his own body to behave the way he wants. The fact that other guys are in trouble couldn't matter less to him. *The University of California's Wellness Letter*, a monthly publication, listed the following conservative percentages: by age fifty-five, 18 percent of men report the problem; by age sixty-five, the figure increases to 30 percent; and by the age of seventy-five, 55 percent of the male population report suffering from impotence. I'm dead certain the numbers are on the low side. But not all of them want to kill themselves."

"Maybe they're senile and can't remember what it was for?"

The doctor smiled gently, "No, I think that when a lucky man has a vital woman in his life, one who simply adores him, she understands that when he's happy in bed, she's happy, too. You'll only make yourself miserable if you pre-decide that you can't start over with another woman and make sparks together. Sex is a life-giving force, as robust and unstoppable and instinctive as breathing. Working with impotency is nothing more than a challenge."

"So you're saying that if you have the right partner a satisfying relationship is possible?"

"Possible? John, it's where a loving couple gets inventive. Giddy sex is available to you at any age and under any circumstance with the right partner. What I want you to understand is that when two people who are crazy about each other want an intimate relationship, they will find their ways. That's what hands and lips and mouths are for. That's what nuzzling and licking and sucking are about. That's what oils and creams and jellies and rubbing and caressing and all manner of touch can do. Coital sex is only one expression of intimacy—just one, John. Everything's going to be fine. I'm willing to bet the farm on it."

"Easy for you to say. Bet you don't even have a farm," John laughed good-naturedly. He was truly encouraged for the first time in a very long while.

"Look, if you think you'd feel more confident I can set up an appointment with a urologist to check you out. There's the Viagra route, and various mechanisms and surgical procedures as well. For now, however, my advice is to skip that woman into bed as soon as you can and let the devil do his best."

"You sound like some Baptist preacher, Doc."

"Well hallelujah! And that's why you're going to pay big bucks to my secretary on your way out. Now get yourself out of here and let some really disturbed soul have your chair."

◆ ◆ ◆

And the days flew by ... Before John knew it, he and Eric were waiting at the airport for Alice's flight to clear its passengers and luggage, John and his son stood where they could watch two possible entry doors giving onto the concourse where Alice might come through. "Dad, this is so cool. Forty-five years—it's so hard to believe—forty-five years go by, then you go out and buy a book, and with the help of phone and computer and fax, we find her in twenty-four hours!"

"If this visit goes the way I'm hoping it will, I'm going to send Culligan—the guy who wrote the book—a nice fat finder's fee."

"That'd probably be a first. You know, there's something I'm curious about—you never told me what it was like, the actual separation from Alice. How did it happen?"

It was a scene etched in memory for John. Peel back the years and he was seventeen again, he could still feel the hurt and the disbelief at his parents' wall of silence, his standoff with his father in the driveway as a moving van pulled away and his life and dreams began to disintegrate. The scene remained clear in his head; the years fell away ...

"Dad! Tell me, for gawdsake, what the hell is happening here?"

"Just get in the car, John. And you can stop swearing."

"I don't get any of it! How can you do this? I left the house at nine o'clock this morning to meet Alice in the park—we're both leaving for college in six weeks; there's a lot to decide. Four hours later I arrive home to find a moving van pulling out of the driveway taking everything we own, you tell me, to *California*? Dad! What in hell is going on?" John was beside himself.

His father didn't answer him, didn't look him in the eye; it seemed all the man could manage was a puny shake of his head as he turned away. The dull sound of the heavy oak front door closing seemed to punctuate the end of their life in Tennessee.

John watched in utter confusion as his mother crossed the front porch with her head down, shamefaced, and her black taffeta evening coat wrapped tightly around her as if to hold herself together. She made her way toward the car, awkwardly navigating the graveled drive in skinny satin party shoes. She was still wearing the clothes she wore to cocktails at the club the evening before. He knew she'd been crying; she looked totally defeated. He waited for her to explain, but she, too, shut him out and climbed into the front passenger seat of the Desoto without a murmur.

"Christ, this is some kind of a nightmare. What's wrong with both of you? I'm not going to California. I'm not going anywhere at all without some answers."

"The car, John, now. I will not have your insubordination. Just get in, don't make it any worse than it is."

They passed Alice's house on the way out of town. Her mother was at the curb opening their mailbox, and John frantically tried to roll down the window and call to her, but his father sped up, and his mother slunk further down into her seat.

The drive from Tennessee to California seemed longer to John than his entire seventeen years of life. He had no money in his pockets, and his parents wouldn't give him any to call Alice. They drove nonstop with the windows up, car and passengers existing on gas and ham sandwiches wrapped in wax paper. Every hundred miles his parents switched turns at the wheel without exchanging a word. His mother appeared to be freezing and continued to wear her taffeta wrap even as the temperature soared the further west they went, and she simply stared ahead when John asked her to roll down her window for a little air.

A silent holocaust of three days and nights driving in demoralizing silence was broken only occasionally by a sob and shudder from his mother, the cause of which was left unexplained; his father's face remained fixed in despair. John's father spoke once to tell John that there would be no explanation or discussion ever over the sudden decision to move across the country.

"What about college?"

"Pack up your dreams, son. No college." At John's father's words, his mother whimpered like a whipped dog and slumped forward.

"I think Mom fainted!"

"Then she's the lucky one." That was in Texas; his father stopped speaking altogether in Texas.

Heartbroken at the abrupt turn of events, his parents' wall of silence, his total perplexity as to the whats and whys of leaving Chattanooga without any sane reason, John gave up trying to speak to either of his parents. He wanted badly to hear Alice's voice; he wanted to hold her close. He mostly slept; it was easier than being awake in the overheated car as he sank further and further into an unreachable space where he didn't ask anything of his parents or expect anything from them. A change in personality can happen at the speed of sound.

John felt his own son's steadying hand on his shoulder. He blinked and shook his head slowly to clear his long-ago memory and said simply, "I wasn't withholding my history, son, but it's important to understand the times, to understand that forty-five years ago a parent's authority—my father's decision, in this case—governed. Such a thing would never happen in today's world. The future that Alice and I talked about incessantly could never have been destroyed by parental decision. Young people today claim the right to their own decisions over family position or opposition, and I'm all for it."

A woman's voice on the scratchy PA system announced, "Flight six o two from Memphis will exit through gate four. Pasajeros del vuelo numero seis zero dos de Memphis saldran por la puerta quatro."

John took a huge breath and grinned shakily at his fantastic son, "Oh hell, this better be the smartest thing I've ever done." John, nervous and excited, and his son, practically as nervous, waited in "Arrivals."

◆　　◆　　◆

As Alice waited for her bags with the rest of the passengers from her flight, she felt like she was about to jump out of her skin. On the two-hour flight, she'd talked the ear off her seat-mate with the story of her first love. She told him how she and John had been inseparable all through high school and about the shock of his family's sudden departure the summer after their senior year, six weeks before they were to leave for medical school.

"The day they left town, John and I spent the morning in the park, and he said nothing about his family's plan to move. I was heartbroken and couldn't understand why he didn't write or call to explain what happened. From that day until ten days ago, I'd heard nothing from him, and that day was forty-five years ago. Isn't it wild?"

"Didn't anyone know where they'd gone? It's pretty hard for three people to disappear without a trace."

"I think his father arranged the departure so there were no loose ends, no unpaid bills or unsettled contracts, no forwarding address. At the time there was whispered gossip about his mother, a scandal involving her and the married manager of the club we all belonged to, but grown-ups stopped speaking and shushed one another when I came near. No one would tell me anything, but I overheard my mother telling a lady on the phone that it was a good thing the Ludlows got out of town before the club asked for his mother's resignation."

"No one talked?"

"Not to me. I pretty much stayed in my room and cried. I was utterly miserable. At first I spent most of my time imagining terrible ways to end my life and writing long letters to John that I couldn't mail without an address. Then it was time to leave for college, and my attitude changed. I got mad. That entire first year at med school I went to lectures, studied long hours, ate, slept few hours, and was rude beyond belief to any guy that was nice to me. Any boy who asked me out was cut dead—there was no way a man was getting close to me again."

"Being hurt and lonely—it had to be devastating."

"Eventually I got tired of being angry and rejoined the human race. There was an air force base nearby and I met a terrific guy who was stationed there. We married soon after I graduated. Bone cancer caused his death in his early fifties."

"After all the emotional turmoil you went through when John disappeared, why would you even want to have anything to do with him now, much less see him?"

"My mother died a year after my husband died. I hadn't spent much time with her since I'd left home; her misplaced morality was difficult for me to accept. When I returned to Chattanooga to settle the estate and go through her things, I found three hundred sixty-six unopened letters from John stored in two cardboard cartons in her attic. She was probably afraid to destroy them. They were dated every day for a year from the day of his arrival in California."

"The letters explained what happened the last day I saw him, the grim car trip across the country, his own heartache and longing for me, and his decision to write daily for a year hoping against all odds that I wouldn't give up on him. It hadn't occurred to him at the time that my mother was grabbing his letters out of the mailbox and hiding them from me. All my life I remember her always being at the end of the driveway waiting for the mailman to come by."

"John wrote that he'd tried to phone several times but that my mother always answered the calls. At first she told the operator to say that I wasn't home, later that I didn't want to speak to him and to not call again. A few weeks later our old number was disconnected, and the new unlisted number wasn't given out by a telephone operator. My mother thrived on gossip and mentioned frequently that gossip had never tainted her family. God deliver me from Southern women!"

"What did you do? Did you let him know that you'd found his old letters?"

"No. For starters I didn't know where he was. What I did was try to find him through an excellent professional agency that specializes in finding lost friends and relatives. They found him for me, all right, but I stopped short of calling him when they said he was married and had a son."

"Then came the absolutely amazing phone call ten days ago from John. Do you think for almost every woman there's someone she once loved so strongly that she's never quite forgotten what it was like? A person whose memory won't go away?"

"Perhaps for each of us there's an unresolved romantic ideal from our past quietly awaiting attention. Do you ever wonder what life would have been like if he hadn't left town?"

Alice flashed him one of her signature wide-mouthed smiles as she pulled her small case from the moving luggage carousel, "That's why I'm here. Only this time I plan to stick around until I find out for real."

John knew her in an instant. The same glorious sparkling eyes and generous smile. He spotted her the second the double doors opened—she almost flew through them straight into his wide-apart arms and hugged him as though she planned to never let go again. She let out a shriek when she caught sight of his son over John's shoulder. "You're almost exactly as I remember your dad!" Alice giggled in surprise. "And almost as handsome!"

"What do you mean "almost"? I'll tell my wife you were mean to me," Eric was laughing at his father's unmistakable joy at holding an equally radiant Alice.

Alice stepped back to look John straight in the face. "And you! You're not planning to leave me in another park for forty-five years, are you? Because I was hoping maybe you could come up with a better idea this time around."

"Oh, Allie-Alice, I'm full of better ideas," his face was alive with pure happiness as he hugged her right back. "I'm betting the farm on this one!"

42

How to Get Invited to Parties

Are you ready to start going to parties, but it hasn't happened yet because no one's invited you? Now what?

Here's the big clue: you get invited to parties by giving parties that everyone will remember.

If it's a sit-down affair, a party can be as many people as the number of chairs you own. Stand-up parties should be no more than twenty people if you really want to spend some time with each of your guests. Or it can be the most people you can cram into your house if it's a pay back affair and it seems a great idea to have everyone at once.

Man or woman, when you're new at this business of entertaining on your own, a good start is to invite two or three friends together for supper once a month or once a week. Everyone is flattered to receive an invitation. Be smart and don't have the same group together all the time. Conversation becomes entirely predictable, and viewpoints get to be so expected that the gatherings become boring. So shake up that guest list—change it often to include single men and women you've just met as well as old acquaintances. A fireman, a professor, a country singer—the most unlikely people can interest one another, often because of their differences. Nothing is more boring than eight lawyers en masse. Or eight nutritionists.

A recently divorced woman who presently has less disposable income might edge away from entertaining altogether if she's worried about finances. But it's not necessary to spend a lot of money to entertain nicely, and it's dumb to spend a lot of money if you don't have a lot of money. The idea is to have fun, not to go into debt; apple cider in crystal stemware is as festive as champagne.

Keep in mind that entertaining doesn't always have to involve shopping, cleaning, and cooking. Tea in a city museum courtyard, a long, chatty brunch of brown rice bowls and Asian salads at a health food eatery, or an earlier-than-usual breakfast at a retro-diner if you're inviting a working pal is good. Even if you're on a limited budget you're not going to get stuck with a bar tab over a plate of blueberry waffles at seven thirty in the morning, nor are you apt to get in big financial trouble treating a friend to a glass of wine in a snazzy deco bar followed by a free jazz concert in the park. A visit to the zoo monkey house followed by lunch at the zoo cafeteria can also make for a fun outing. Good company and rare settings are the ingredients of a happy memory.

One thing that will ensure a single woman or man a place on other people's party lists is if you throw the kind of fun parties with interesting guests that everyone is dying to be invited to—that alone will keep your social calendar full. It further increases your popularity when, in attending other people's parties, you don't make it a practice to down a snootful of whiskey and then try to down your host.

43

Find Your Personal Neighborhood Escape Hatch

It's one of those evenings when you just have to get out of the house or you'll go raving mad. You're home alone, unpleasantly restless, and nothing's working for you. The last thing you want is to call a friend and spread your nervousness, and the idea of paying bills, writing letters or reading or watching TV holds zero interest. But where can you go at nine o'clock at night by yourself?

It's a real dilemma: your nerves are screaming, you're determined to go somewhere, but you can't think of one place where you'd feel comfortable on your own that late in the evening.

You need an advance plan to cover this exact kind of situation, an already mapped-out bolt-hole to head for on the spur of the moment. The idea is to line up a place in your neighborhood where you feel entirely at ease walking in at any time of the day or night. It can be a restaurant/bar that stays open late. It can be a local pub or a jazz club. In order to feel that you can go there at any given time and be recognized by sight, if not by name, you have to make it part of your life well ahead of crisis time. You want to find a friendly spot where someone familiar will start up a conversation or ask you to sit with him, or her, or them: in other words, a cozy neighborhood hangout. Don't wait until you hit an evening where you feel so desperate for company that you might take off in your car and end up frustrated and in tears at some totally inappropriate disco full of twenty-year-olds or redneck drunks. That's just asking for headaches.

When you are alone again for the first time in years, there may be days when you feel terribly lonely, dispirited, and uncomfortable in your own skin. Your mood spirals downward, and the road ahead seems to stretch impossibly uphill. Even if it's been a few years since you lost your partner, you still hit the odd time when your stamina fails you. And this is where you have to be smart and create safeguards to counter a bout of unwanted solitude.

Forlorn feelings of defenselessness can be occasionally overwhelming, but if you've paved the way by carefully choosing a friendly local pub that serves meals as well as drinks, where you'll find expected faces, perhaps a billiard competition or a dart game in progress, it can be your escape-hatch. You know the people by name who work the bar and serve the usual crowd, you and some of the regulars have a little history of banter and past laughs. Make a habit of dropping into it on a weekly basis either with friends or solo so you'll be okay to head there on your own when you reach one of those absurd times when stress has built to discomfort level.

In a large city, it's especially important to cultivate your own comfort areas, including smaller family-run grocery stores, a friendly dry cleaner, a favorite fruit and vegetable market, a fishmonger, a bakery, a butcher shop, and a popular diner that you frequent. The neighborhood becomes your territory, a small chunk of the city where you recognize and smile at young mothers wheeling their babies in strollers, the kids on skateboards, the man at the corner newsstand where you buy your lotto tickets on the weekend. You can run into the shoemaker at the post office, and have him tell you that your boots are stitched and ready for you. Or the lady at the convenience store tells you that your friend, Stuart, was in ten minutes earlier and said if you came in to tell you he was headed to the café for blueberry pie. You can't avoid feelings of aloneness; after all you *are* alone presently, yet it doesn't have to be a permanent state of mind, by any means, if you are prepared to do whatever you can to help yourself. The choice to be happier is always yours, and it helps to become close to people who need you, too, as a good friend.

44

Home Stagers: a winner job for a creative entrepreneur

Home stagers are a little known but growing breed of professional whose job is to enhance a home's marketability. As a home stager, you will consult with house sellers and suggest improvements and small changes to maximize the sale price of their property in a competitive real estate market.

It can be a simple sale where a couple is moving into another house and doesn't have either time or inclination to upgrade their home to realize a better profit. However, there are many other reasons a house might be up for sale: a couple is breaking up, and the house must be sold and the profits divided, a widower's grown children have married and left home, and the place is too big for him alone. Or a seller's husband died, and the widow wants a new start in fresh surroundings. A divorced man or woman wants to move into a condo and forget the hassles of maintaining a property alone. The various conditions of a sale often leave one single-again woman and/or one single-again man presently unattached. Good to know.

Most of these house sellers have long lost that quick interest to improve the house they've lived in for a while, but now want to sell at top dollar. And here's where you, the stager, come in to dress up their house for successful resale; with your efforts the house rises in value, which pleases the seller and returns money to his pocket, the broker's pocket, and to your pocket. Everyone wins.

This is how it works: Register a business name and design a smart business card. Decide on a reasonable consulting fee that is refundable only if the job is contracted. Next you contact different real estate offices and let them know that if they list a dowdy-looking or messy, overcrowded house for sale that you are available, for a fee, to clean up the mess, get rid of aluminum window blinds, polish windows, strip and refinish floors, hang curtains and pictures, even upgrade a kitchen or bathroom where doing so will return a higher profit at point of sale. Your fee can range from $1,500 for a dowdy condo that simply needs cleaning, de-cluttering, and a bit of perking up with colorful cushions, curtains, and area rugs, to a much higher fee depending on the amount of work and size of the house. You will get rid of worthless junk and store items such as mismatched furniture and personal collections (perhaps an entire wall's worth of trophies and framed blue ribbons from dog shows) that distract buyer interest; by minimizing the clutter, the full space and capacity is visible. When the work is completed the restyled house will have universal appeal and sell faster in a slow market and at a higher price in a fast market.

Home stagers are also known as fluffers, house primpers, house dressers, house tweakers, or resale decorators. Do you see yourself as a professional stager? For a creative person who loves improving houses and organizing garage and basement clutter, this is an ideal money making occupation with built-in opportunity to meet new people. While the interior of the house is extremely important, much of your work will focus on the outside of the house. Curb appeal of any property is crucial, as a smart exterior is a huge draw for would-be buyers. It is the first and last picture that will remain in the mind of every potential buyer.

When you remove an ugly aluminum screen door that presently obscures a handsome raised-paneled front door, the house immediately increases its value. The next thing to eliminate is any indoor-outdoor stair and porch carpeting; whoever dreamed up that kind of floor covering should be sent to stand in the corner wearing an idiot cap.

Lawn and borders need to be trim. The addition of lushly planted flower boxes attached to front window ledges, exterior lights with clean glass globes, simple house numbers, and freshly painted steps will further invite potential buyer appeal. Strategically placed potted trees at either side of a front door and at the base of front steps will lend an air of generosity to the home's entrance.

The enormous popularity of home makeover programs on TV has resulted in buyers who expect more for their money, yet not everyone who hopes to sell a house has the time, vision, or talent to effectively achieve a look of sophistication that appeals to today's homebuyers. Not everyone has the ability to blend fabrics and furniture styles with taste. If you have this kind of know-how that can raise the value of a house with small improvements, home staging is a fun job tailor-made for you.

Home stagers indulge their creativity to improve property; they also put some cash in their pocket and make new friends in the process. So far it sounds like one grand idea!

- *FABJOB.COM, an Internet site, has information on other types of work that have no age limits and that do not require exceptional training. Personal shopper (for busy or confined clients), party planner, and mystery shopper (where you get paid to shop in stores or eat in restaurants and submit reports on service to the management) are a few that are named.*

45

Expand Your World With Computer Savvy

At the supermarket where I shop, there's a fabulous-looking man, probably about sixty-nine or seventy, with a deep baritone voice, a full head of crinkly steel gray hair, his own strong white teeth, and this devilish grin that just dares sassiness from the customers. One evening after he'd bagged my fruits and vegetables at the checkout counter, he asked, "Can I get you and your groceries to your car?"

"Sure. You can walk me to my car—you can walk me home if you'd like," I told him, a broad smile on my face. Actually I thought it was a swell idea, even if I pretended it was a joke.

"Hey! Feels good to get outside; the fresh air smells great. I've been in that damned store since noon."

I was feeling pretty nervy so I plunged right in. "Would you do this job if you had some training that allowed another kind of work?" I broached the subject while he was loading groceries into my car trunk. I wanted better for him.

But instead of taking me seriously, he shook his head emphatically, laughing blatantly at my words till he saw my embarrassment and touched my arm in apology.

"No way I want another job! I co-anchored the evening news for CBC in Toronto for twenty-five years, and long ago I decided that when I retired or was booted out—whichever came first—I'd do something with absolutely no pressure, no deadlines, no producers, no directors, no prima donnas, no makeup to wear in front of the camera, no jet lag, and no sucking up to sponsors at contract time."

"Migawd. For one of the very few times in my life I'm speechless!"

"I think it was kind of sweet that you wanted to help me."

"Oh, please. What I wanted was to whip you into shape."

"Hey, not everyone has a retirement job of first choice. I'm one of the lucky ones." He had me laughing at his zany logic.

But he's right, there. Not everyone does have a retirement job of first choice.

A lot of older men are doing yard work and handyman jobs or bagging groceries at the local supermarket for extra cash or simply because they can't stand retirement and want something to do so they won't go clear around the bend. However, retired people too often *are forced* to accept these jobs because they are not computer literate, and unskilled labor is about the only area of work open to a person without computer skills. It has nothing to do with lack of intelligence; it has everything to do with having held positions that for years didn't require use of that particular technology.

Computer literacy is needed in most jobs today. And if you don't already have that ability, learning to use a computer is yet another way to gain self-confidence. It will get your mind working in new directions that will at first frustrate you beyond belief, but later lead to a terrific sense of accomplishment.

You didn't grow up with computers so it's nuts to plead dumb, but if you sign up for a computer course and apply yourself to learning a new-to-you technology, you'll be placing yourself in a highly desirable category for employment. Plus it opens up another social path as you become friendly with your classmates and teachers over the weeks of your computer training.

Every day thousands of mature singles take advantage of a number of learning opportunities and gain ground with increased self-reliance. A self-confident man or woman is someone everyone wants to be around. The special feeling that comes from achieving a new skill, from putting an idea into practice and knowing that you are capable, is its own reward. And if you turn your new knowledge into a part-time job, your self-confidence will turn cartwheels.

Aside from the satisfaction of conquering a new frontier, you'll learn how to send e-mail, enter "chat" rooms on the Internet, and "meet" other Net users with similar interests, hobbies, or problems. You can research medical information, make airline and restaurant reservations, dermatology and dental appointments, and look for a used car to buy or a new person to date. Computer savvy expands your world.

Even if having a job is the last thing on your to-do list, and not anywhere near what you want to do with your time, it's still a huge thrill to master a computer. It's a machine, for heaven's sake, it's not your enemy, and one of the nicest things about being able to handle it is that it bridges a generation gap and allows you to stay in close touch with youth. It's important also to be considerate when you learn to use e-mail: ask your friends if they want to be on your mailing list to receive forwarded jokes, prayers, chain letters that must be sent to twelve others before sundown or something dire will befall them, and other useless stuff. Many people do not want to be on such a list. Actually, most people delete those messages.

46

Flattery Is a Win-Win Situation

It's practically impossible to flatter a man too much. What man is going to object when you look at him wide-eyed and say, "You are positively amazing!" or, "What a brilliant observation! I never thought of it in quite that way; I think you're positively a genius," or, "Who but *you* would have thought of that? I absolutely treasure the way your mind works."

What do you say? Is that over the top for most guys? It is not.

Later on, as the relationship deepens, don't confine your flattery to his flamboyant mind. Move on to his peerless knees and his tight butt, even if it has ridges deep as moon runnels. He'll love it, and probably think you didn't notice any imperfection. The thing is there's a big difference between not noticing, and choosing not to pay any attention to, things that aren't apt to change.

You have to be truly besotted with him to carry it off, but you can make almost any man of any age believe that you are his sweetest darling if you're prepared to play the flattery game with him. Men, let's say 99 percent of them at a low guess, do believe implicitly in their own luster. Besides, it's fun to flatter!

When he's off visiting his children and grandchildren, send him tabloid-type letters to feed his fantasies. Talk about his body parts in ways that glorify and exaggerate (it's fun to talk a little hoodlum occasionally). Don't worry on this one—give it to him good! He'll love it, and so will you. Also it'll prime his pump for answering your letters in an equally exciting way. His trip will quite likely be cut short.

Never forget it—any woman who understands how to flatter men has heaps more fun in life. You'll get a lot more attention and receive many more invitations from your man, and get a whole lot more dirty looks from parade-drenching women who are apt to say to the same man, "Good heavens, don't tell me they still let *you* drive at night!"

Grooming for all your Fabulous Tomorrows: Part Five

47

Who Said Younger Is Better? (For Women Only)

What's wrong with a woman dressing to suit her age? At sixty, why do some women try to look thirty?

You see older women all the time at the supermarket or walking around the mall in short shorts, miniskirts or stretch pants—clothing that's designed mainly for kids, but when worn by older women to subtract years, it adds them instead.

What's great about trying to look like a teenager? Teenagers look weird. They know they look weird. They're supposed to look weird. Weird is their badge of honor. However, leggings and ankle bracelets on a sixty-five-year-old are in the same category as combat boots and tight-fitting striped sweaters—that of "Holy cow! What were you thinking!" Some older women need to consult a sharply lit full-length mirror.

On one hand it's great that older women today decide in favor of being vibrant and youthful in their outlook. It's wonderful to find women who feel fresh and funny and young-minded, but if they keep dressing younger and younger, pretty soon they're going to be running around in their christening dresses, and you never see that on Internet dating profiles, do you—"Handsome sixty-nine-year-old widower seeks widow or divorcee sucking on a pacifier"?

This country is obsessed with youth. A seventy-year-old woman continues to wear makeup and do her hair in the same style she wore at the age she remembers as being the most glamorous time of her life.

Thick jet eyeliner flipped at the outer corners, frosted blue eye shadow, and eminently skippable ice pink lipstick—ridiculously dated makeup that makes an older woman appear older, not younger. Ice pink lips look more corpselike than alive, and very dark lipsticks also don't work on older faces.

The worst hair mistakes for older women are usually home-colored, home-permed, shoulder-length rivers of curls that start at the scalp and quit at the split ends. Or gray hair colored a harsh black—that choice is hell. Neither one does an experienced face any favors.

All hair-coloring kits (especially the kits with the streaks) should come with warnings for older women: "Don't try this at home ... or anywhere else." Instead, how about any woman over fifty treating herself to an appointment at the best hair salon she can afford?

Splurge! Pretend that a fabulous haircut and superior color is well worth the price of a new Mercedes, and that anything slightly less than that is very fair.

Be sure to get the colorist to write down the formula of the new tint so it can be repeated at your next appointment, or for you to take on vacation or to another less-pricey salon.

Find recent copies of *Vogue*, *Style*, and *Elle* fashion magazines at your local library. Study them carefully and plan a well-designed wardrobe from what you see that will suit your life and your activities. It's not necessary to buy the designer labels in the fashion layouts; it's just to get ideas of shapes, simplicity, hem lengths, and colors. A good place to start is to invest in a basic black lightweight wool crepe suit, an off-white silk shirt, a black leather handbag, and black leather pumps with a medium heel. You'll never go wrong when you stick with quality fabrics and classic lines, understated, never flashy. Underneath you can be wearing a frothy aphrodisiac from Frederick's of Hollywood. Who's to know?

With a classic suit as a foundation to your wardrobe, you can add different scarves, sweaters or shirts, belts, necklaces, or showy lapel flowers to change your look. However, bright eyes and a warm smile are, without question, the best accessories of all. Your dentist should play a big part in your good looks, too.

If you're unsure of your clothing choices, perhaps you know someone who has a certain style that you admire. Is there a man or woman friend you can ask to help reconstruct your wardrobe? Maybe even go shopping with you? Different people have different skills, and most people feel flattered to realize you want their advice. A simple rule is stick to classic style in main pieces and use accessories to follow trends.

You also want to look good when you're home alone; it feels good to dress up even when you're not going out. You know for a fact that you feel better when you look your best; that includes makeup, earrings, and no more slopping around in jeans and old house slippers.

You want to look better than good. Being your own age is something you can't avoid, but taking pride in looking marvelous at any age is aiming high, and you'll love the results. Your family will love the results also, and so will someone you are about to meet who may become a new friend and/or love interest.

48

Who Said Younger Is Better? (For Men Only)

It's very true that women do love being around a man with a youthful outlook and a sense of humor, but is any good-looking older woman attracted to a man who presents himself as a teen-ager? Think about it. Most women, who have brought up a family of real children, are not in the least interested in having an aging boyfriend who dresses like he's a perpetual kid. Leave the ponytails, bare feet, cutoffs, hole-in-the-knee jeans, baseball caps, and low-slung baggy pants behind with the teenagers where they belong. And that also includes older men in trendy clothes from Banana Republic; just get rid of all the acid-washed denim clothing you may own, as well as earrings, sleeveless tank tops, and *anything* mesh!

Then there are the men who seem to be surgically attached to cell phones *wherever* they happen to be—in a car, on the street, or in a restaurant. What do you think—impressive? No. That's kids stuff. It's also a big bore to hear grown men use phrases such as "that's cool, man" or "what's goin' down, dude?" Not only because they sound like jerks, but even teenagers no longer use those expressions. Most women can recognize a desperate man at a glance—which means any insecure man who needs to be thought of as young when he's not, or kid-scruffy when he's collecting social security checks and should know better. A grown man with low self-confidence holds no serious appeal for women.

If a woman were offered a choice between a handsome man and a confident one (there's no reason a man can't be both, of course, but for arguments sake, let's say she had to choose), there would likely be no hesitation whatsoever. There's something gloriously seductive about a mature man who is self-confident, who isn't trying frantically to appear younger or straining to hold back the clock.

A self-confident man is like a magnet to most women. It's important to the majority of women to feel a sense of solidness in her mate; an aura of power is the strongest of all aphrodisiacs. Power in a man is nothing more than simple, sure strength of character. She wants a man who is his own person, who doesn't pretend to be someone or something he's not.

Who said younger is better? Not so. A self-confident man of sixty, seventy, eighty is probably better looking now than he was at age twenty-five, especially if he's achieved a satisfying measure of success in his life. Think of some of the most appealing older actors around today. Who are they? Why do they still exude sensuality?

They are the confident, well-groomed, well-tailored, clean-shaven, positive thinkers without a chip on their shoulder. They are well informed on politics and world affairs and generously make time for important causes. They are actors by profession, but much more than mere role players in their personal lives. Robert Redford created the Sundance Film Festival to showcase the work of younger independent filmmakers. Christopher Reeve, the original star of the Superman films who was left paralyzed after a horseback-riding accident, worked tirelessly until his death to raise funds for spinal injury research. Placido Domingo opened a school for young tenors to help further budding operatic careers; he coached their voices, he didn't try to be one of the boys. Have a look at the strong paintings of an older Anthony Quinn or the novels of Gene Hackman. Did Tony Bennett resort to rap or try to ingratiate himself with new kids on the charts? No, but he encourages young talent, and they all want to perform with him publicly. When he's done his stint, he gets off the stage. He's not trying to be their best buddy. Paul Newman gives his time and cash to support his Hole in the Wall Camps for handicapped kids around the country. The recipe for respect is intelligence, humor, talent, self-confidence, and generosity.

Interesting men find it unnecessary to use the jargon of youth or to dress like kids. They own their age; they are the men who will never outlive their attractiveness. What's more, they are the men women want.

49

Bald and Faking It

Are you pretending not to be bald? There should be a booby prize that goes to all men who comb long strands of hair over a bald spot. Some highly intelligent guys do it; you're not the first. Apparently it has little to do with brains. But it's really dumb because every woman alive who knows anything about men is well aware that a bald man is infinitely more charismatic and sexy than a man with a cock-eyed hairdo.

You cannot truly believe that no one notices that nothing's growing underneath the combed-over hair. You know there are no actual roots that produce hair on the top of your head, and, I have to tell you, in a high wind it looks like a couple of snakes are doing a belly dance over one ear. On a calm day it looks more like a grocery store bar code plastered to the top of your head.

Think of the king of Siam. Yul Brunner made a career out of hairlessness, don't you know, and women were cuckoo about him! American women dreamed about that hairless brute—maybe not enough to go and look after his eighty children, but obviously a bunch other women did.

Do not turn the page. I'm not done with you yet. Your wife has been gone for a while now. You're single again, and you're in charge of your own appearance; the carefully placed hairs on your balding head only make you look foolish.

You can, and I hope you will, do yourself a huge favor—spring for a decent haircut! Then watch out for the ladies giving you the eye.

50

Behind Closed Doors

When it comes to personal grooming habits, the trick is in knowing which will intrigue your new love and which will be visibly off-putting.

You want to keep your new relationship romantic from the get-go. Even if your past marriage was considered ideal by any standard, you know there are certain attitudes and habits to overhaul if you want your new love to stay starry-eyed for a long long time; you have a fabulous opportunity right now to start fresh.

Keep most personal grooming practices behind closed doors. Absolutely solitary. These are not romantic procedures to witness.

Here's the **don't** list:

- No flossing your teeth as you watch TV with your partner.
- No sitting around with plastic curlers in your hair or clipping your toenails when you're together.
- No tweezing chin hairs or plucking your eyebrows when you're in the same room.
- Coloring your hair is another turn-off. You are both aware you don't have true sun-kissed blond streaks; it doesn't need illustration.
- Spooking out your new love with the aspect of a facial mask and fresh cucumber slices on your eyelids isn't cool.
- No toothpick action allowed in front of your new mate.
- Do not remove your partial plate from your mouth unless solo; gargle *alone*.

Your new love-interest doesn't truly believe that your appearance is completely natural, but it's fun to promote the illusion. Hey, if any of us went around totally natural, we'd be in big trouble. After a number of decades of living, anyone over fifty years realizes that "natural" just doesn't cut it.

There are exceptions. Some grooming procedures will fascinate your new love and offer the assurance of exclusive intimacy:

- A very feminine woman will intrigue her man by brushing her hair at her vanity table dressed in a pretty robe or asking him to brush it for her. A spritz of perfume on her wrists, low on her bare back, and behind her knees allows him a glimpse at some of her wiles.

- A distinctly masculine act for a man is to secure a bath towel around his waist, apply shaving cream on his face, and shave in front of the bathroom mirror, all the while grinning at his lady-love sitting on the edge of the tub. A playful dab of foaming cream on her nose will have her smiling a knowing smile. Best of all, writing her name inside the shape of a heart on a steamed-up mirror will have huge rewards.

Bring it on! You're Ready for a Brilliant Future: Part Six

51

A Mate-Selection Quiz for Late Lovers

What have you gotten, or what are you getting, yourself into—a solid relationship that has every chance to succeed? Or trouble? The questions in the quiz are designed to make you think. There is no pass or fail. The questionnaire is definitely not a test paper to take along on a first date.

Here we go!

1. When did you meet? Did you meet through common interests? Through friends? Through an arranged introduction?
2. What did each of you do before you met?
3. How long were you on your own before you met?
4. Are you happier single? With a live-in partner? With a steady partner who lives apart from you? Or married to the one you love?
5. Before you met did you make a conscious decision to find a new love?
6. How did you go about it? Did you have a plan? A list of requirements or qualities you wanted to find in a future mate?
7. After you first met and talked, was there an exchange of phone calls, cards, letters, e-mail, gifts, or flowers? Who gave first, and who gave back?

8. Do you think it important to have one mate be the leader, the decision-maker, the protector? Does it matter to you which one it is as long as you're both comfortable?

9. How soon after you met were you interested in each other as future mates?

10. When you met were you in your fifties, sixties, seventies, or eighties? Is there a difference in your ages? And, if so, was it a factor in your decision to choose one another?

11. Was religion an issue?

12. Is one of you religious, the other agnostic?

13. Did you ever consider living together without marriage in mind?

14. Were there doubts or struggles along the way that had to be resolved?

15. Were they resolved to your satisfaction?

16. If applicable, how long after you met did you marry?

17. If married, did you have a marriage contract? Do you both have updated wills reflecting your current spousal situation? Do you have a living will that covers all possibilities of incapacitation?

18. How much discussion was there before you married about separate financial responsibilities within the marriage? Is either of you a big spender? Is one of you frugal, or cheap? Who's the best tipper? I'm Canadian, and there's a piece of wit that says that the difference between Canadians and canoes is ... canoes tip! It's my guess that this is a lot funnier if you don't happen to be Canadian.

19. How do you rate yourself as a partner, a husband or a wife now, compared to yourself as a partner in your first marriage?

20. Is your present relationship easier or harder? Less or more dramatic? Are there fewer or more tears over a disagreement?

21. Is either of you jealous of the other? If so, how does it affect the marriage? Do you feel jealousy is connected to caring? Or to immaturity?

22. Do either of you manipulate the other?

23. Do either of you feel you could do with less instruction from the other? Less being told what to do, when to do it, or what you should have done if you hadn't done what you did do? Do you think one should be committed to the marriage or to the marriage partner?

24. Do you enjoy each other's company and have wonderful adventures together?

25. Were either of you working outside the home when you met? Does this continue to be the situation? Do either or both of you work in a home-based office? Is it a good arrangement?

26. Do you each have a room or a space you can call entirely your own?

27. Are you intellectually compatible?

28. Did either of you relocate to be together? Do you live in a home that either of you owned before you met? Or did you make a fresh start in a new place for both of you?

29. Did either of you have pets? Was/is it a problem?

30. Do either of you smoke? Does this cause argument?

31. How does your day-to-day housekeeping work? Do you share grocery shopping and household chores, cooking, washing dishes, organizing doctors' appointments and the like? Do you share in arranging your social life—planning dinner parties and trips, writing thank-you notes and returning phone calls?

32. How much time do you spend together privately? And separately? And together with friends and/or family? Do you have time to comfortably pursue your own dreams?

33. How does your new mate treat service people (e.g., waitstaff in restaurants, cleaning help, salespeople in stores)?

34. Do you have similar tastes in TV programs (e.g. C-SPAN vs. sit-coms), restaurants, sports events, art, newspapers, music, theater, books, movies? Does it matter?

35. Are you in agreement politically?

36. Do you have close friends who don't get along with your new spouse or partner? Is it a problem? Is it better to enjoy one another or please every old friend?

37. Do either or both of you have adult children? How often do they visit, and for how long?

38. Are you in agreement about the length and frequency of visits from relatives and friends, and do you tell visitors in advance how long they can stay?

39. Do your children like or resent your choice of a new mate? And how about your spouse's children—do they like you? What did you do right or wrong to bring this situation about? How do you handle the situation, or do you ignore it?

40. If your children don't trust your new husband (or wife), how do you handle it? The children of the partner with the most money are usually the most critical. Does that apply here?

41. Do the two families of adult children get along well? Or politely? Or explosively? Does it matter? Are there resentments that bother either of you over your adult children's attitude? Do you visit your family (siblings and children) as a couple or separately? What about traditional holidays?

42. Who does the driving when you're together in a car? Why?

43. What do the grandchildren call each of you? Is there any animosity from grandchildren as a result of either of you supplanting their natural grandparent? Is it a good or bad idea to have your spouse's grandchildren call you grandpa or grandma?

44. This has no place whatsoever in the quiz, but it's a peeve of mine: personally, I can't stand the word "grandmother." I tell my own grandchildren that each of them has his or her own name, and so do I. I do not call the oldest of my grandsons "Grandson number one," and the next, "Grandson number two." Nor do I call my beautiful granddaughters "Granddaughter number one," "number two," "number three," and "number four." So why should they call me the generic name of "Grandma" when I'd rather they use my given name—it is my name, after all. Now when they introduce me to friends they say, "This is my grandmother. Her name is Pat, and you can call her Pat."

45. Is your new mate in any way an embarrassment to you? Crude language? Sloppy personal grooming? Poor manners? A bit of a snob? Fragile ego? Pushy? Cheap? Spoiled? Talks nonstop? Is your mate's speaking voice well modulated? Abrasive? Does it bother you?

46. In your opinion, are the two of you emotionally mature? Is either of you a critic? A controller? Judgmental? Narcissistic? Defensive? Bossy? Bad tempered? Often testy? How serious is it? After an argument, who is the first to apologize and mean it?

47. With regard to finances, are either of you worried about money? Okay? Comfortable? Or very comfortable?

48. If your mate dies before you do, will you have to move? What would change for you?

49. Did you get what you wanted in this partnership? Has it been emotionally satisfying? Do you have fun together when you're by yourselves?

50. Do you look out for each other? Do you feel safe with your partner? Has there ever been any physical abuse at any time? How about mental abuse?

51. Do either of you put the other one down with sarcasm or cruel remarks? Are demeaning remarks, couched as clever wit, made in front of friends and family about your personal appearance, your cooking, your housekeeping, your tardiness, your intelligence, or your spending habits? Do you speak up about how it makes you feel?

52. Did you act too soon in this relationship? Any regrets? Would you do it over again, knowing what you now know? What would you do differently if given the chance?

53. Did your parents have a warm relationship? Did either of your parents remarry?

54. How about your general health? Pretty good? Anything serious for either of you? Any deafness? Forgetfulness? Depression? Heavy drinking? Obesity? What effect has it had on the relationship? What does each of you see as your own most irritating habit, and do you have intention or hope of reforming?

55. In what month was each of you born? What was your birth order in your original family?

56. Who cooks? Why?

52

Good-bye Loneliness, Hello Happiness

Kumar, a sixty-seven-year-old widower from New Delhi, India, gives do-it-yourself workshops at a Home Depot store. Hannah, at seventy-two, has been widowed for two years. She decides to attend the free workshops and learn how to make flower boxes for two front windows of her home; she's attracted to the enthusiastic instructor. Having lived all her life on a farm in rural Kansas, she's never met anyone so exotic. At a second session, designed to teach the group how to wire a lamp, Kumar keeps an eye on all the do-it-yourselfers, but he spends most of his time by Hannah's side helping her with her project. They each spend a lot of time smiling at one another. He asks her to come to his next session on faux finishes. Can this pair be a match?

Ruth is a quiet, shy widow of sixty-four. She works with tarot cards and reads fortunes three days a week in the mall. One afternoon she meets Peter, a seventy-year-old divorced, extroverted used-car salesman, in front of the meat counter of a specialty food store. The two of them have a long wait as the butcher prepares Ruth's crown roast. Peter's entertaining antics have her giggling like a schoolgirl when he tells her how he cooked his first steak in Latvia; laughing at himself, he pushes up his sleeves and demonstrates how he scrubbed the bloodied meat with household cleanser before he boiled the steak in a pot of salted water. Ruth says, "You should either write a cookbook or be a stand-up comic; I'm not sure which." Happy in her company, Peter carries Ruth's groceries to her car and asks if he may call her. What kind of chance does this accidental meeting of two opposites at a meat counter have for romance?

Jonathan, a divorced gifted seventy-one-year-old choir director, is at the ballpark to watch his beloved granddaughter, Annie, in the batter's box for the Special Olympics baseball game. He stands on the sidelines of the field next to Liz, a sassy-mouthed widowed seventy-six-year-old hairdresser, as she cheers on her adored grandson, Gavin, also a Down's syndrome child. Gavin is the pitcher for the same ball team. After the game Jonathan and Liz take the two excited kids to McDonalds. Usually any woman Jonathan dates is uncomfortable around his precious granddaughter, but not Liz, who is clearly enjoying herself. Are their common interests in two very special grandchildren enough of a start for long-term interest in one another?

Joyce decides to do a freelance video shoot of Anthony Detroit, the handsome African American mayor of a nearby town, whose growing popularity is attracting political attention. Her camera catches his interaction with the smiling crowds at a Fourth of July public picnic. He definitely notices her shoulder-length blond hair and striking Dutch good looks, and acknowledges her with a wave and a big hello from the podium. After his speech, Joyce watches him from the cold drinks stand as he searches for her in the crowd. She decides to keep him wondering about her for a little longer, a week should be about right. She knows he'll be speaking at a Girl Scout rally on the following Saturday and plans to be there with her camcorder. Joyce came to the United States from Holland five years earlier and is the owner of a popular beach motel; at forty-eight, she is a recent divorcee who lives in the next village. Anthony, the dynamic mayor who retired at sixty from the metropolitan police force, is a widower of two years. Does this combination have positive possibilities?

Marla, a sixty-three-year-old Asian bank teller, went out of her way to be sympathetic and kind to Aaron, an eighty-year-old bank customer whose wife was terminally ill with cancer. When Aaron did his banking he always went to her wicket; he found her gentle manner and wisdom comforting. Marla sent him a card after his wife's death. Two years later these two got together when Aaron spotted her in a street crowd at a St. Patrick's Day parade and was so glad to see her again. The seeds for that romance were planted long ago by her kindness.

Marylou is the widow of an intellectual zoology professor who'd had, for his entire career, a very narrow range of interest in the physiology of the Gobi desert camel, in particular its hydrating and water-retention systems. She plowed through forty years of that kind of talk. Once he was gone, Marylou, at sixty-nine, was looking for someone whose company and conversation she liked a lot better. Yorghis, a fifty-nine-year-old Greek widower at the garden center, listened carefully to her plan for a rock garden, helped her choose the best plants for her hillside rockery, delivered the flats, worked alongside Marylou digging in the soil, and loved the iced tea breaks while they sat on her porch and traded stories of their very different childhoods. They worked together contentedly on Yorghis's days off throughout the summer. Think this match has a future?

They *all* have a good chance to succeed. Give them time to develop.

In each of these cases, both the men and the women were open to new experiences with unexpected people. Ask yourself what it is that you really want. You've been married before, or you've had a long time partnership with someone and, if you have a family, your children are no longer children. This is your time. You are the star this time around. Whoever you choose as your next partner in life has to please just one important person: *you.*

You no longer have parents to please. Your children may not be in love with the person you choose as your new partner, but they have their own lives and most likely no longer live in your home. It is not up to your family or friends to approve your choice. By now you've learned a lot about yourself and about what and who gives you pleasure. Your values are deeply rooted. Your new mate can be from a different country, have a religion other than yours, be a different skin color, or speak another language. The only true requirement is that you find someone you love to be with, someone you absolutely love loving, someone who, in turn, makes you very, very, very, very happy.

And only the two of you can make the possibility of a beautiful relationship a reality.

Bibliography

AARP (American Association of Retired Persons). Google their site for information.

AARP Legal Services: free consultation for members. www.aarp.org/Isn4.

AFP (The Association of Financial Planners). Google their site for information.

Americans United for Separation of Church and State, Washington, D.C. Google their site.

Behrendt, Greg, and Liz Tuccillo. *He's Just Not That Into You.* New York, N.Y: Simon and Schuster, 2006.

Berlitz International Inc. Over 400 language schools worldwide. www.berlitz.com

Brown, Steven Kerry. *The Complete Idiot's Guide to Private Investigating.* Indianapolis, IN: Alpha Books, 2003.

Caldron, Paul, D.O. 2007. Age Erasers for Women/Arthritis (Internet information). *Rodale boo*k Edit id 7.

CARP (Canadian Association of Retired Persons). Google their site for contact information.

Carper, Jean. *Food: Your Miracle Medicine.* New York, N.Y: Harper Collins, since 1993 with perennial updates.

Classmates.com: a resource to find old school friends.

Copper Canyon, Chihuahua, Mexico al Pacifico Railway. Google their site for information.

Cruises.com: for all shipping lines cruise information.

Cruiseshipjob.net: the biggest cruise ship staff hiring body in The United States.

Culligan, Joseph J. *When in Doubt, Check Him Out.* Miami, Florida: Hallmark Press Incorporated, 2001.

Dartmouth University Alumni Tours. Google for tour information.

Delinsky, Barbara. *Uplift: Secrets From The Sisterhood of Breast Cancer Survivors.* New York, N.Y: Washington Square Press, 2003.

Diener, Ed, and Martin Seligman. 2005. The Science of Happiness. *Time Magazine* Jan. 17.

FabJob.com: publishes career guides.

Feng Shui. *The Complete Idiot's Guide to Feng Shui*: Amazon.ca

Fung, Dr. James. Pettibon system: info@absolutehealthclinic.com

Greenwald, Rachel. *Find a Husband After 35.* New York, N.Y: Ballantine Books, 2004.

Haan, Dr. Mary N., MPH, PH. 2003. Is Cognitive Decline Inevitable? *Neurology Reviews.com* Vol.8, No.10.

Habitat for Humanity Web site: habitatforhumanity.com

International Cooking School Vacations. Google their site for course information.

Kalish, Nancy. *Lost and Found Lovers.* New York, N.Y: William Morrow Publishers, 2005.

Mensa: www.mensa.org: information on the high IQ society, and free intelligence tests.

National Shared Housing Resource Center. Google their site for information.

Nuckols, Dr. Cardwell C., and Bill Chickering. *Healing an Angry Heart.* Oakland, California: New Harbinger Publications, 1998.

Paikin, Steve, journalist-host and moderator of TVO's *The Agenda.*

Peterson, Jordan, professor, clinical psychologist. 2007. Plasticity of the Brain. *The Agenda, TVO* April 12.

Rosenberg, Daniel, and Richard Kirshenbaum. *Closing the Deal.* New York, N.Y: Harper Collins, 2005.

Soas, Dr.Amir. 2007. Creating New Brain Cells. *Discovery Health Newsletter:* July 11 issue. Soas, Dr. Amir. 2000. Read, Read, Read. *HEALL (Health Education Alliance for Life and Longevity) Publications* August issue.

Statistics Canada (Statistiques Canada) www.statcan.ca: 2006–2007 statistical information and summary tables in English and French.

Thomset, Kay, and Eve Nickerson, featuring complete medical information by Donald H. Holden, MD. *Missing Words.* Washington, DC: Gallaudet University Press, 1993.

Train travel Canada: Google for current excursion information.

Train travel in the United States: Google for current excursion information.

United States Bureau of the Census Web site for statistical abstract 2007, population tables.

University of California's Wellness Letter, monthly publications. Apply online.

Vitiello, Michael V. Ph.D. 2006. Special Report by Bob Condor. *The Seattle Post-Intelligencer* Feb.20.

Worldwide Volunteer Vacations. Google their site for information.

978-0-595-43825-9
0-595-43825-3

Printed in the United States
100835LV00003B/109-126/A